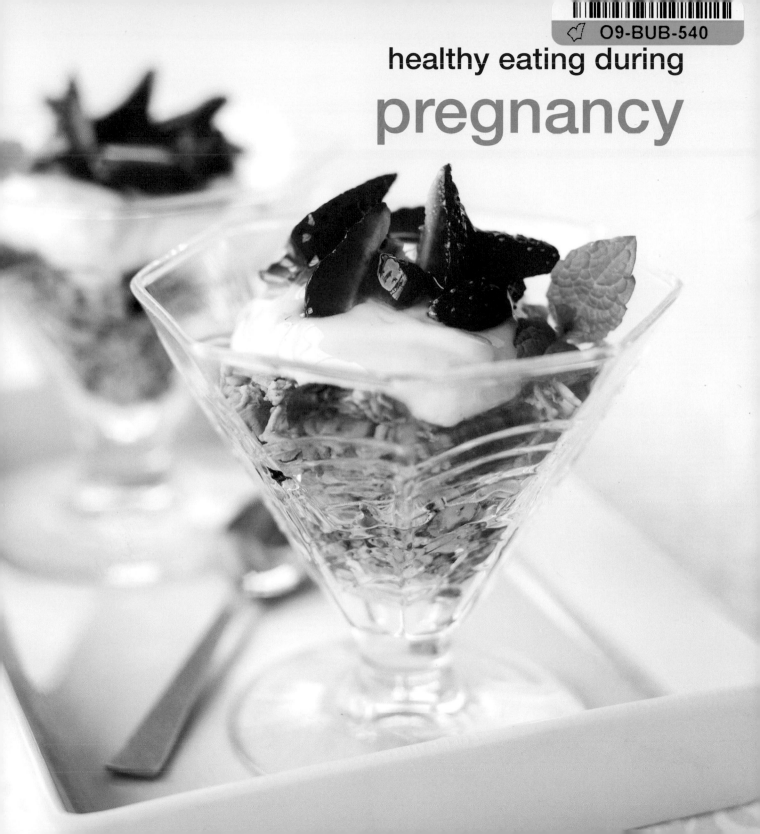

healthy eating during
pregnancy

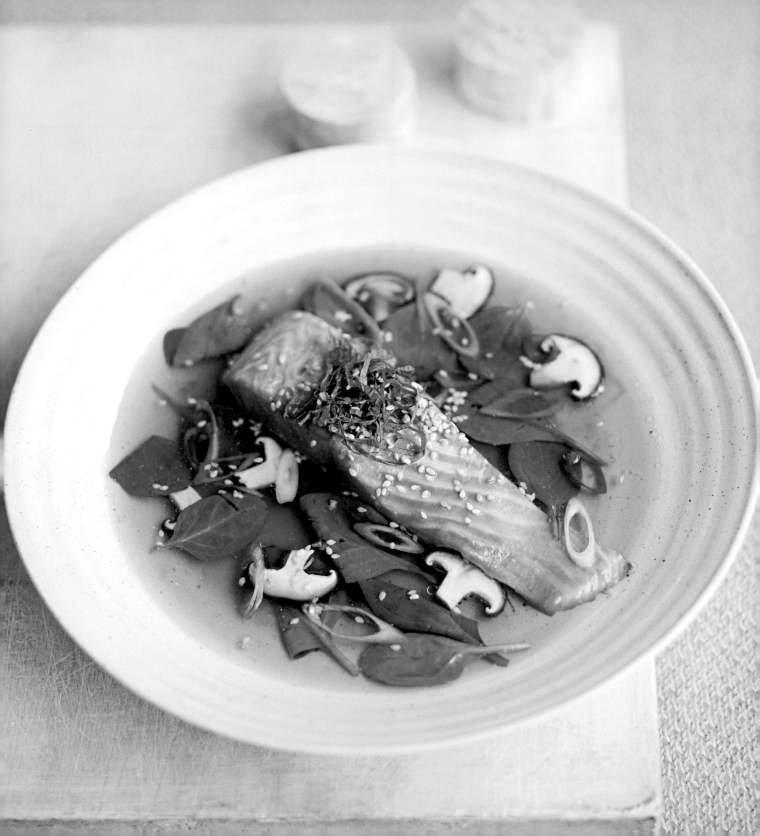

Erika Lenkert
with Brooke R. Alpert MS, RD, CDN

healthy eating during
pregnancy

Photography by Will Heap

Kyle Books

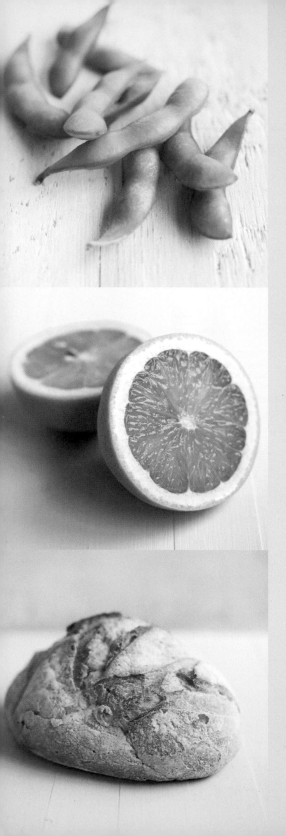

Published in 2011 by Kyle Books
an imprint of Kyle Cathie Limited
www.kylebooks.com

Distributed by National Book Network
4501 Forbes Blvd., Suite 200
Lanham, MD 20706
Phone: (800) 462-6420
Fax: (301) 429-5746
custserv@nbnbooks.com

Project editor Anja Schmidt
Designer Geoff Hayes
Photographer Will Heap
Food styling Aya Nishimura
Prop styling Wei Tang
Copy editor Jane Tunks
Production by Nic Jones, Sheila Smith and Lisa Pinnell

Library of Congress Control Number: 2011922333

Color reproduction by Sang Choy
Printed and bound in Singapore by Star Standard Industries Pte. Ltd.

contents

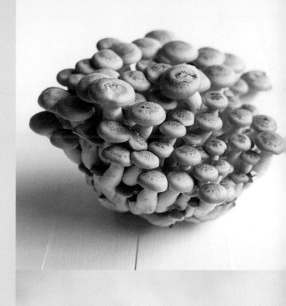

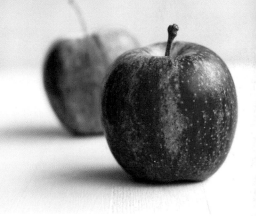

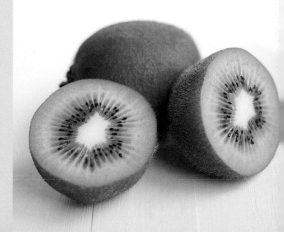

foreword by HealthyWomen

As the executive director of HealthyWomen, the nation's leading independent health information source for women, I have monitored the comings and goings of new research, health trends, and dietary fads for nearly 20 years. And, as a registered nurse in maternal and fetal health, I have witnessed the one issue that remains a constant: the expectant or new mother's desire to do what is best for her child.

In *Healthy Eating during Pregnancy*, Erika Lenkert and Brook Alpert have undertaken the daunting task of separating fact from fiction when it comes to eating for two and providing modern-day solutions to pregnancy cravings, best eating practices, and healthy weight guidelines. Breaking down the science behind nutrition and defining nourishment needs in layman's terms, the authors give clear and concise advice for all stages of pregnancy and postpartum recovery.

As an active member of the healthcare industry and an ardent advocate for women's wellness education, I believe that a commitment to healthy eating now will only edify your baby's wellbeing and nutritional balance for their many years ahead. According to a WomenTALK survey conducted by HealthyWomen in 2010, only one-quarter of women surveyed understand their role and influence on their child's risk of becoming obese, and that risk starts during pregnancy.

HealthyWomen's mission is to inform and empower women to make smart health decisions and *Healthy Eating during Pregnancy* does just that. It provides a nutritional roadmap that—if followed—will help keep you on the road to wellness and get your baby off to the best start possible. As women, we are the gatekeepers of food in most of our homes and understanding the influence that we have on our family members can never be learned too early, or even too late.

I know that an expectant or new mother wants to do what is best for her child, and now you have a tool to help you do just that. Put your plans into action with *Healthy Eating during Pregnancy* and your child will thank you for it…of course, you'll have to get through those toddler, 'tween, and teen years first!

In good health,

Elizabeth Battaglino Cahill, R.N.
Executive Director
HealthyWomen

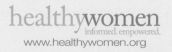

healthywomen
informed. empowered.
www.healthywomen.org

introduction

If you have this book in your hands, congratulations! Not only are you pregnant, but you are also doing one of the smartest things you can do to ensure the health and happiness of you and your unborn baby. Why? Because, as you've probably already discovered, pregnancy comes with a cornucopia of dietary conundrums, from what you should or shouldn't eat to how much weight you should or shouldn't gain to how on earth you can possibly stay on track when your cravings are strong enough to make you consider breaking into a bakery after-hours. Add to that the litany of boring pregnancy-food recommendations out there (tofu nut loaf, anyone?), and it's enough to make even the nutrition-conscious mom-to-be shrug her shoulders and dive into a tub of ice cream.

That's where this book comes in. The following introductory information, provided by the fabulous nutritionist and mommy Brooke R. Alpert, answers all your nutrition questions and provides concrete guidelines for smart eating for all nine months. Then I follow up with 100 spectacularly delicious, even downright indulgent, recipes that make eating for optimum baby and mommy health a truly satisfying experience. Collected from some of the world's finest chefs and my own kitchen, you will be making these fast and easy-to-prepare dishes for years to come, especially once your little one starts to move past rice cereal.

So don't be afraid to cater to your newly gargantuan appetite, even if it's peppered with hurl-inducing bouts of nausea (hey, we've got food for that!). With these recipes, you can actually have your cake and eat it, too.

Just remember to eat three small meals a day and two snacks, which will help ward off hunger attacks and keep your body energized for the miraculous task at hand. Supplement with prenatal vitamins as directed and enjoy a variety of foods, ensuring you get a wide variety of essential nutrients. Beyond that, just savor this time—literally and figuratively. With all the hard work your body is doing, you absolutely deserve it.

Warmest regards to you and your growing family,

Erika Lenkert

eating for two

Though we'd all like to believe that "eating for two" literally means doubling up on calories and dessert helpings, that's not actually the case. Here's why: The average woman needs to consume between 1,800 and 2,200 calories per day to keep her engine running smoothly and efficiently, and a normal, healthy, full-term pregnancy requires an approximate 80,000 additional calories over the course of 40 weeks, or 280 days. That's a mere extra 285 calories each day, or a total daily caloric intake of about 2,500 calories per day. Very active women and teenagers may need as many as 2,900 calories per day and should ask their doctors for caloric guidance.

But before you go planning a two-desserts-diet, consider this: You don't even need extra calories during the first trimester, when the baby's developmental focus is on the brain, not the brawn, and recent guidelines in the United Kingdom advise that even during the third trimester, when your baby is seriously bulking up, only 200 extra calories are necessary.

On the bright side, as we mentioned earlier, it is recommended that you eat five—you heard us, five!—times each day. While we're not talking heaping platefuls of food, calorie-minded guidelines offer plenty of room for dining pleasure, as evidenced by the sample diet plan on page 10. Eating frequent portion-controlled meals and snacks ensures you don't get overly famished—a surefire way to bring out the beast in even the most gentle pregnant woman—and your developing baby gets a steady flow of much-needed nutrients.

what to gain?

The optimum amount of weight to gain during pregnancy depends on how much you weighed prior to becoming pregnant as well as how many children you are carrying at one time. A woman at a "healthy" prepregnancy weight, as determined by the body mass index (BMI) chart opposite, should gain approximately 25 to 35 pounds during her three trimesters carrying a single baby. Targets for women who were "overweight" are 15 to 25 pounds, and it's recommended that women who fall into the "obese" or "extremely obese" category on the BMI index should try to gain no more than 11 to 20 pounds. "Underweight" women should aim for 28 to 40 pounds to help prevent having a low birth-weight baby.

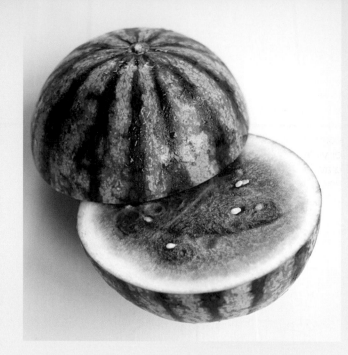

Women with a "healthy BMI" who are expecting twins or triplets will need to gain approximately 35 to 45 pounds. Unfortunately, there is not enough information for women expecting three or more babies, but significant weight should be gained, approximately 2 pounds per week during the second and third trimesters. To see what category of starting weight you fall into and how much you should gain for a healthy pregnancy, determine whether you fall into the "healthy," "underweight," "overweight," "obese," or "extremely obese," category using the BMI chart at right.

when to gain?

Regardless of your prepregnancy weight, there are some healthy weight-gain guidelines that are ideal for ensuring you and your baby are getting enough, but not too much, caloric energy. Keep in mind that these are only guidelines and each pregnancy is unique and weight changes may even vary for the same woman from pregnancy to pregnancy:

During the first trimester, a weight gain of 1 to 1½ pounds per month is considered normal. However, women suffering from severe morning sickness or even all-day sickness may actually lose a slight amount of weight during this time. (And conversely, women who are indulging as if every meal were their last will gain more.) Since every woman is different, it's not critical to be right on target here, but it is important to contact your doctor if you are having a hard time keeping food or water down, as you may be suffering from hyperemesis gravidarum, which is a severe form of morning sickness that needs to be monitored closely. See Morning Sickness (page 23) for more on this.

During the second and third trimesters, your weight gain will begin to pick up to about ½ pound to 1 pound per week.

Some months you may gain more, some less, which is normal with all of the hormonal and physical changes happening (think breasts enlarging as they prepare for milk production, your uterus expanding, the placenta growing, and most importantly, your baby developing). For some women, weight gain slows down during the last few weeks of pregnancy, even though your baby will continue to grow because, as your body prepares for labor, it holds onto less fluids. And if that nesting instinct kicks in, women tend to burn extra calories as they physically prepare for the baby's arrival.

BMI chart

Legend: Underweight | Healthy | Overweight | Obese | Extremely Obese

Weight lbs		100	105	110	115	120	125	130	135	140	145	150	155	160	165	170	175	180	185	190	195	200	205	210	215
kgs		45.5	45.7	50.0	52.3	54.5	56.8	59.1	61.4	63.6	65.9	68.2	70.5	72.7	75.0	77.3	79.5	81.8	84.1	86.4	88.6	90.9	93.2	95.5	97.7
Height in/cm																									
5'00"	152.4	19	20	21	22	23	24	25	26	27	28	29	30	31	32	33	34	35	36	37	38	39	40	41	42
5'1"	154.9	18	19	20	21	22	23	24	25	26	27	28	29	30	31	32	33	34	35	36	36	37	38	39	40
5'2"	157.4	18	19	20	21	22	22	23	24	25	26	27	28	29	30	31	32	33	33	34	35	36	37	38	39
5'3"	160.0	17	18	19	20	21	22	23	24	24	25	26	27	28	29	30	31	32	32	33	34	35	36	37	38
5'4"	162.5	17	18	18	19	20	21	22	23	24	24	25	26	27	28	29	30	31	31	32	33	34	35	36	37
5'5"	165.1	16	17	18	19	20	20	21	22	23	24	25	25	26	27	28	29	30	30	31	32	33	34	35	35
5'6"	167.6	16	17	17	18	19	20	21	21	22	23	24	25	25	26	27	28	29	29	30	31	32	33	34	34
5'7"	170.1	15	16	17	18	18	19	20	21	22	22	23	24	25	25	26	27	28	29	29	30	31	32	33	33
5'8"	172.1	15	16	16	17	18	19	19	20	21	22	23	23	24	25	25	26	27	28	29	29	30	31	32	32
5'9"	175.2	14	15	16	17	17	18	19	20	20	21	22	22	23	24	25	25	26	27	28	28	29	30	31	31
5'10"	177.8	14	15	15	16	17	18	18	19	20	20	21	22	23	23	24	25	25	26	27	28	28	29	30	30
5'11"	180.3	14	14	15	16	16	17	18	18	19	20	21	21	22	23	23	24	25	25	26	27	28	28	29	30
6'0"	182.8	13	14	14	15	16	17	17	18	19	19	20	21	21	22	23	23	24	25	25	26	27	27	28	29
		13	13	14	15	15	16	17	17	18	19	19	20	21	21	22	23	23	24	25	25	26	27	27	28
		12	13	14	14	15	16	17	17	18	18	19	19	20	21	21	22	23	23	24	25	25	26	27	27
6'3"	190.5	12	13	13	14	15	16	16	17	18	18	19	20	20	21	21	22	23	23	24	25	25	26	26	
6'4"	193.0	12	12	13	14	14	15	15	16	17	17	18	18	19	20	20	21	22	22	23	23	24	25	25	26

where the weight goes

Come birth day, you might be surprised to find your baby only weighs 7 pounds when you've packed on enough weight to represent five healthy children. Fortunately, the added weight is not simply new appendages to your thighs, hips, or belly. Between the baby, placenta, amniotic fluid, and breasts, the numbers add up quickly. Alas, beyond bloating from water retention, most additional pounds acquired during pregnancy are mementos of overindulgence. They are also yours to keep—and lose—after your baby is born.

Average weight breakdown

Where	How much?
Baby	6-10 lbs
Placenta	1-2 lbs
Amniotic fluid	2 lbs
Breasts	1 lb
Uterus	2 lbs
Increase in blood volume	3 lbs
Body fat	5 or more lbs
Increased muscle tissue and fluid	4-7 lbs
Total	**At least 25 lbs**

why how much you gain matters

There is more to monitoring weight gain than whether or not you will fit into your favorite maternity jeans after pregnancy. Gaining too much weight can heighten your risk of gestational diabetes (high blood sugar levels brought on by pregnancy), lead to a larger (and thus harder to deliver) baby, and potentially even heighten the risk of your baby being an overweight or obese child and adult.

On the flip side, eating enough or even a bit too much helps ensure your infant will be born at the desirable weight of more than 5.8 pounds, or 2,500 grams, which lowers his or her chances of developing heart and lung disease, diabetes, hypertension, and hypoglycemia later in life. It also lessens the likelihood of a low Apgar score (a test to determine an infant's physical condition) at birth.

2,500 calories a day

If all this talk of caloric monitoring makes you think you're in for a bland, restrictive dining experience for the next nine months, check out this chart highlighting a single day's menu possibilities, complete with recipes from this book.

Meal	Calories
Breakfast	
Zucchini Frittata	154
Two slices whole-wheat toast	180
Decaf skim latte (8 oz)	70
Snack	
Sesame Honey Almonds	210
Nonfat vanilla yogurt (6 oz)	130
Lunch	
Decadent Chicken Soup	135
Deluxe Greek Salad	310
Whole-wheat pita (small)	80
Snack	
Parmesan-Dusted Kale Chips	90
Ginger Limeade	44
Dinner	
Comforting Pot Roast	380
Oven-Roasted Parmesan Fries	376
Chinese-Style Green Beans	63
Dessert	
Chocolate Coconut Oatmeal Cookie	120
Skim milk (1 cup)	90
Total	**2,432**

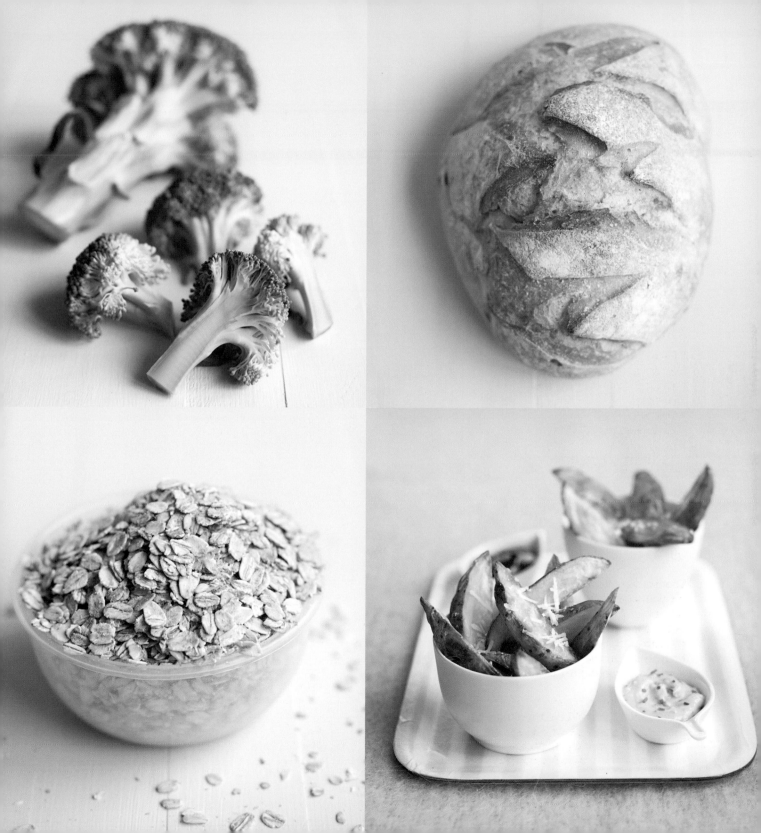

noshing for optimum nutrients

Surely you know that it's not just how much you eat, but what you eat that matters when you're growing a baby. Still, knowing how to identify and consume the most helpful nutrients can be a challenge even to the healthiest moms-to-be. These primers can help you bite through befuddlement and get to the meat of the matter.

macronutrients

All the energy you need for pregnancy comes from your diet—specifically carbohydrates, protein, and fat. Together with fiber, these are the four macronutrients necessary for a healthy pregnancy.

carbohydrates

Carbohydrates are a great source of energy for your pregnant body because of all the possible calorie sources, your body burns them the most quickly and efficiently. The energy supplied by carbohydrates are needed for both you and your baby's brains, muscles and central nervous systems. Without enough daily carbohydrates, your body will turn to protein for energy instead of using it for the important growth functions for your changing body and especially for your growing baby. (For more on protein, see page 14.) As a result, carbohydrates should make up a significant amount of your daily calories. (Need an excuse to indulge in pasta? Now you have it!)

Simple carbohydrates versus complex carbohydrates
Not all carbs are created equal. "Simple" and "complex" carbohydrates have different benefits, and in the case of simple carbs, potential drawbacks.

Simple carbohydrates—found in fruit, milk, and even some vegetables—provide plenty of healthy nutrients, vitamins, minerals, and fiber in addition to energy and are broken down quickly by the body. But they are also found in the form of refined sugars and processed foods, such as sodas, cookies, cake, and candy. These types of simple carbs contain "empty calories," meaning they have no nutritional benefit. Eating too much of them can lead to excessive weight gain, high blood sugar, and even gestational diabetes. Complex

carbohydrates—found in whole grains, root vegetables, beans, and more—contain B vitamins, which aids in the growth and development of your baby. They also contain magnesium, a mineral that helps relax the uterine muscular lining and build bones and regulate nerves for you and your baby. They also contain trace minerals, such as copper, which aid in the formation of connective tissue. Needless to say, complex carbs are very good for you and your little one.

Good Carbohydrates Choices	Carbohydrates to avoid or eat sparingly
Whole grains	Granulated sugar
Whole-wheat bread	Cakes
Potatoes	Cookies
Sweet potatoes	Muffins
Legumes	Pastries
Beans	Candy
Low-fat dairy	Soda
Fruit	
Barley	
Couscous	
Quinoa	
Brown rice	
Multigrain cereal	

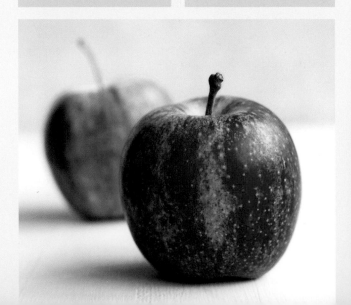

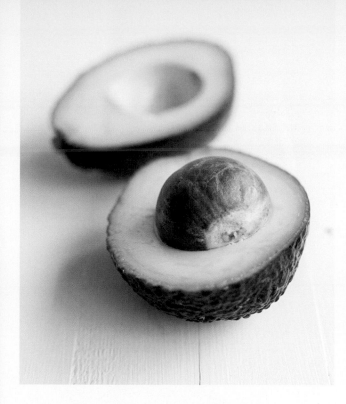

fat

Contrary to what we are regularly told, fat has a lot of important beneficial qualities, especially for pregnant women. An essential nutrient, it helps support the growth of the placenta and other tissues helps develop your baby's brain and central nervous system, prevents preterm delivery and low birth weight, and transports vitamins A, D, E, and K from you to your growing baby. Plus, with the highest amount of calories per gram compared to other nutrients, fat aids in providing enough calories to make sure your body has the stamina to grow your baby and keep you energized along the way.

Add to that the fact that essential fatty acids during pregnancy and lactation have been linked to babies with higher intelligence, better vision, and more mature central nervous systems and you've got all the reason you need to welcome fat as much as 30 percent or less your daily caloric intake.

That said, all fat is not created equal. There are four kinds of fats found in food: monounsaturated, polyunsaturated, saturated, and hydrogenated, and some are better for you than others.

The good
Monounsaturated fat (found in olives and avocados): Considered a good fat because it has a healthy effect on blood cholesterol levels.

Polyunsaturated fat (found in vegetable oils, nuts, and seeds): Contains the good fatty acids omega-3 and omega-6, which are crucial for your baby's development.

The bad
Saturated fat (found in red meat, full-fat dairy, and butter): Considered bad because it may increase cholesterol.

Hydrogenated fat (also known as trans fat and primarily found in processed foods): Used to extend shelf life of packaged foods; can increase your risk of heart disease.

Healthy fat choices
Olives/olive oil
Avocado
Peanuts
Peanut butter
Freshwater fish
Flaxseed oil
Canola oil

Tips for low-fat eating

★ Choose lean meats and skinless poultry
★ Trim fat from meat before cooking
★ Choose low-fat or fat-free dairy products
★ Avoid processed foods as much as possible

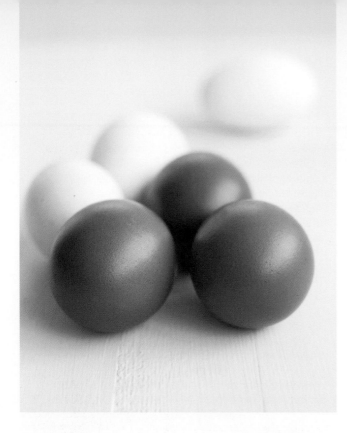

protein

Protein is absolutely critical for pregnant women because it is used to make new cells, manufacture enzymes and hormones, and control fluid balance, which directly affects blood pressure. During pregnancy, more than 25 percent of all the protein you eat goes directly to the baby, placenta, and uterine lining. It also acts as a much-needed energy supply if you don't eat enough carbohydrates.

For the first trimester, your protein intake needn't vary from your prepregnant days. It's during the second and third trimester, when the baby undergoes the most rapid growth, that your protein requirements increase from the daily recommended 50 grams to 60 grams per day. Meeting these needs is very doable—even for women with food aversions, morning sickness, or vegetarian or vegan lifestyles—because protein is present in an amazing array of foods, including grains, nuts, and beans.

There's an extra perk in eating protein: Many foods that contain it also include other important nutritional powerhouses. For example, lean red meat, chicken, and seafood are all great sources of protein as well as iron. Milk, another protein provider, also has vitamin D and calcium, which are important components for bone development.

Alas, some proteins can be high in saturated fats (hello, ice cream, fatty steaks, and chicken skin!), and thus should be consumed in moderation. You can avoid eating the bad with the good by choosing lean meats, skinless poultry, low-fat or fat-free dairy.

Protein-rich foods

Food	Serving size	Protein (grams)
Beef, extra lean, cooked	3 ounces	25
Bread, whole-wheat	1 slice	3
Bulgur, cooked	1 cup	6
Cereal, bran flakes	¾ cup	3
Cheese		
Cheddar	1 ounce	7
Low-fat cottage cheese	1 cup	28
Part-skim mozzarella	1 ounce	7
Chicken, cooked, no skin		
White meat	3 ounces	27
Dark meat	3 ounces	23
Egg	1 large	6
Egg white	1 large	3
Garbanzo beans, cooked	1 cup	18
Lentils, cooked	1 cup	17
Milk, whole or skin	1 cup	8
Peanut butter	2 tablespoons	9
Pork loin, cooked	3 ounces	26
Salmon, cooked	3 ounces	22
Tofu, raw	½ cup	10
Wheat germ	¼ cup	7
Greek yogurt	1 cup	20
Yogurt, nonfat fruit	1/3 cup	7

fiber

Fiber is a cholesterol-reducing component of plant foods that is found in whole grains, vegetables, fruits, legumes, nuts, and seeds. For pregnant women, one of fiber's best benefits is that it can relieve constipation and hemorrhoids (common pregnancy side effects) because it softens and stimulates stools and allows for them to be passed more easily.

An important partner to fiber is fluid. Fiber absorbs a significant amount of fluid while traveling throughout your digestive tract so it's important to be properly hydrated in order to benefit from fiber as much as possible (see Hydration on page 22 for more).

A good amount of fiber to aim for every day is 20 to 35 grams. See the chart below to find out how much fiber is in your healthy food choices!

Fiber-rich foods

Food	Serving size	Fiber (grams)*
Fruit		
Raspberries	1 cup	8.0
Pear	1 medium	5.5
Apple	1 medium	4.4
Strawberries	1¼ cup	3.8
Banana	1 medium	3.1
Orange	1 medium	3.1
Figs, dried	2 medium	1.6
Raisins	2 tablespoons	1.0

*Can vary depending on brand and size

Food	Serving size	Fiber (grams)*
Grains, cereal & pasta		
Spaghetti, whole-wheat, cooked	1 cup	6.2
Barley, pearled, cooked	1 cup	6.0
Bran flakes	¾ cup	5.3
Oat bran muffin	1 medium	5.2
Oatmeal, cooked	1 cup	4.0
Popcorn, air-popped	3 cups	3.5
Brown rice, cooked	1 cup	3.5
Bread, rye	1 slice	1.9
Bread, whole-wheat or multigrain	1 slice	1.9
Legumes, nuts & seeds		
Split peas, cooked	1 cup	16.3
Lentils, cooked	1 cup	15.6
Black beans, cooked	1 cup	15.0
Lima beans, cooked	1 cup	13.2
Baked beans, vegetarian, cooked	1 cup	10.4
Sunflower seed kernels	¼ cup	3.9
Almonds	1 ounce (23 nuts)	3.5
Pistachio nuts	1 ounce (49 nuts)	2.9
Pecans	1 ounce (19 halves)	2.7
Vegetables		
Artichoke, cooked	1 medium	10.3
Peas, cooked	1 cup	8.8
Broccoli, boiled	1 cup	5.1
Turnip greens, boiled	1 cup	5.0
Sweet corn, cooked	1 cup	4.2
Brussels sprouts, cooked	1 cup	4.1
Potato, baked	1 medium	2.9
Tomato paste	¼ cup	2.7
Carrot, raw	1 medium	1.7

*Can vary depending on brand and size

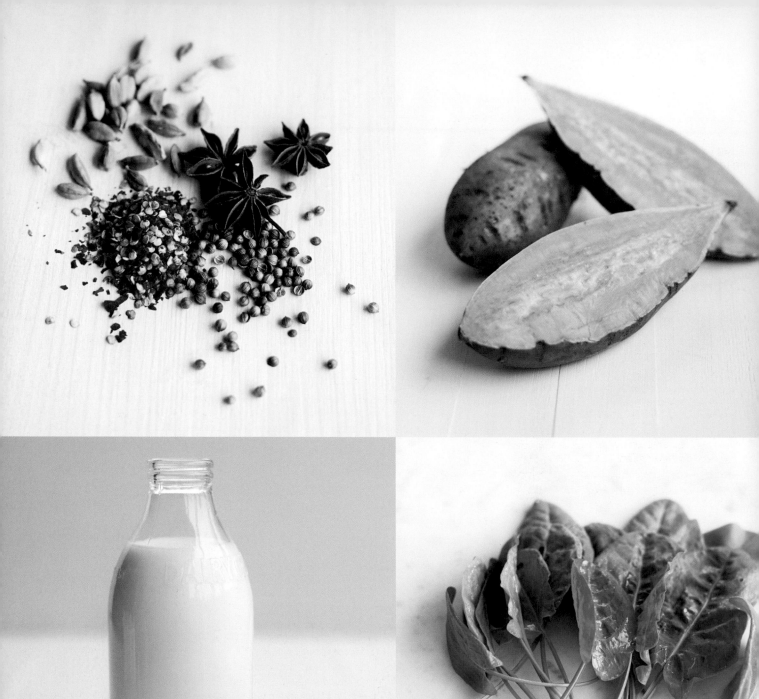

micronutrients

As the name suggests, these nutrients are little guys compared with the "macro" carbohydrates, fat, protein, and fiber. But that doesn't mean they are any less significant. Vitamins, which are technically micronutrients, control your digestive system and the metabolism and absorption of carbohydrates, protein, and fat. Following are some micronutrients that are especially beneficial to you right now.

calcium

Calcium plays a large role in female and fetus health. Circulating through your bloodstream, it is critical for cellular functioning, nerve transmissions, and a healthy heartbeat. Stored in your bones and your body, it is tapped to help build your baby's bones and teeth.

Luckily, your body is so smart that once it recognizes your baby is using up your stored calcium supply, your hormone levels change to allow for more calcium absorption from the foods you eat. This system is so efficient that while pregnant, you may absorb twice as much calcium as you did before pregnancy. However, even heightened absorption doesn't promise you will get enough calcium. The fact is, each pregnancy puts you at a higher risk for osteoporosis later in life, which results in brittle bones that are more susceptible to breaking.

For that reason, it's recommended that pregnant and nursing women get 1,000 to 1,500 milligrams of calcium a day. Many pregnant women take prenatal supplements, which contain calcium, but it's still very important to get enough calcium in your diet.

Dairy products are great sources of calcium, and they also contain protein and vitamin D, which also benefit pregnant women. If you are lactose intolerant or a vegetarian, there are many plant foods or enriched foods that provide calcium as well. However, not all plant foods help your cause. Some foods, such as whole-grain bread, beans, seeds, nuts, and grains, contain phytic acid or oxalic acid (found in spinach, collard greens, sweet potatoes, and beans), which prevent the calcium in that food from being absorbed by the body. To make sure you get enough, look for calcium-fortified foods.

Calcium-rich foods

Food	Serving size	Calcium (mg)
Dairy products		
Milk (all types)	1 cup	300
Swiss cheese	1 ounce	270
Mozzarella cheese, part-skim	1 ounce	185
Cottage cheese	½ cup	75mg
Ice cream	½ cup	85
Non-dairy products:		
Tofu (fortified)	½ cup	260
Soy milk (fortified)	1 cup	250-300
Orange juice (fortified)	¾ cup	225
Salmon, canned	3 ounces	205
Broccoli	½ cup	45
Okra	½ cup	50
Orange	1 medium	50

B vitamins

Because B vitamins help your body release and use energy derived from the food you eat, they are critical during pregnancy. Fortunately, they are easy to come by. Aside from fruits and vegetables, B vitamins are found in most food groups.

Still, because different types of B vitamins perform different functions, you'll want to make sure you graze with variety in mind. For example, thiamine, which is found in pork, whole grains, and enriched grain products, helps release energy from carbohydrates. Meanwhile, riboflavin, found in dairy products, organ meats, and enriched grains, helps your body produce that energy. Niacin works on your general metabolism and is found in meat, poultry, and seafood. B6 vitamins help create cells from protein and are found in poultry, fish, pork, and bananas. B12, which is found primarily in animal products as well as some fortified foods like soy milk or cereal, aid in the body's manufacturing of red blood cells. B12 also helps the body utilize the energy from fat and carbohydrates.

Another B vitamin, folate, or folic acid, is so important for general health as well as pregnancy that many foods are fortified with it. Folate is responsible to producing and creating new red blood cells. A deficiency can lead anyone to a blood disorder called megaloblastic anemia, while a deficiency during pregnancy, especially during the first trimester, can result in a baby with neural tube defects (NTDs), including serious birth defects such as spina bifida and anencephaly. Studies have shown that if all women consumed the recommended amounts of folate before and during early pregnancy, up to 70 percent of all NTDs would be prevented. Studies have also shown that women who take a folic acid supplement for at least one year before they conceive significantly reduce their risk of giving birth to a premature baby.

Folate is found naturally in foods, and folic acid is a form of folate used in fortified foods and supplements. It is recommended that all women of child-bearing age get at least 400 micrograms of folate or folic acid a day either from food (fortified or natural) and/or supplements. Pregnant women should aim for at least 600 micrograms per day as soon as they know they are pregnant, with 400 micrograms coming from a supplement or fortified foods since it is in the more readily absorbed form.

Naturally occurring folate foods	Serving size	Folate (mcg)
Chickpeas, cooked	1 cup	160
Lentils, cooked	1 cup	358
Peas, cooked	1 cup	101
Spinach, cooked	1 cup	263
Strawberries	1 cup	26

Fortified folic acid foods	Serving size	Folic acid (mcg)
Bread	1 slice	40
Oatmeal, instant	½ cup	80
Pasta, cooked	½ cup	100–120
Ready-to-eat cereal	⅛ cup	100–400
Rice, cooked	½ cup	60

iron

Your iron needs double, from 15 to to 30 milligrams (mg) per day, during pregnancy and there are plenty of reasons why. First, your growing baby needs a lot of oxygen to develop and iron is responsible for making hemoglobin, which is the protein in your red blood cells that carries oxygen to your baby. Iron is also a component of myoglobin, a protein that supplies oxygen to your muscles for collagen, a protein in bone, cartilage, and connective tissues as well as many enzymes. Finally, as if iron weren't enough of a nutritional superhero already, it also helps you maintain a healthy immune system.

Considering that your iron needs increase so much during pregnancy it's no wonder so many women experience iron-deficiency anemia when their babies' iron needs increase during the second trimester. Fortunately, many prenatal supplements contain iron. Unfortunately, supplements often cause constipation, nausea, or both, so it's important to eat foods that are naturally high in iron, too. That said, if you are vegetarian or simply having a hard time eating meat during your pregnancy, it's a good idea to consume vitamin C-rich foods with your meals, which help increase iron absorption. Another tip: Avoid drinking coffee or tea with your meals as their polyphenols (chemicals found in plants) can affect your body's ability to absorb iron.

Iron comes in two different forms, heme and non-heme. Heme iron, found primarily in animal products, is better absorbed by the body. Non-heme iron is mainly found in plant foods, and is absorbed less, which is why vegetarians and vegans may need iron supplements.

Iron-rich foods	Portion size	Iron (mg)
Heme		
Beef, tenderloin, cooked	3 ounces	3.1
Beef, sirloin, cooked	3 ounces	2.9
Chicken, skinless breast, or dark meat, cooked	3 ounces	1.0
Tuna, canned	3 ounces	1.3
Shrimp, cooked	3 ounces	2.6
Pork, lean, cooked	3 ounces	1.0
Non-heme		
Fortified breakfast cereal	½ cup	2-9*
Spinach, boiled	½ cup	3.2
Potato, baked	1 medium	2.8
Enriched rice, cooked	½ cup	1.2
Raisins	⅓ cup	1.1
Kidney beans, cooked	½ cup	2.6
Whole-wheat bread	1 slice	0.9
Pumpkin seeds	⅛ cup	4.2
Lentils, cooked	1 cup	6.6
Prune juice	1 cup	3.0

*Depending on brand

sodium

Extra water weight may not be desirable for the pregnant figure, but the fact is that sodium, a component of salt that's also found in food additives, provides more than just swollen ankles. It aids in maintaining the body's water balance, and consequently is critical for healthy blood pressure. So when your blood volume increases a whopping 25 percent during pregnancy, sodium helps maintain normal blood pressure, and aids in muscle contraction and nerve conduction.

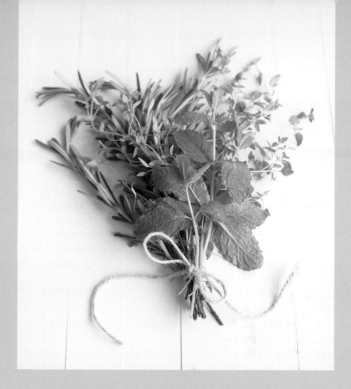

Most pregnant women have no problem meeting the minimum requirement of about 570 milligrams per day. In fact, most consume way more than they need since the nutrient is ubiquitous in processed and prepared foods. To get the benefit without the bloat, aim for 3,000 mg of sodium per day and read nutrition labels of packaged foods to make sure they aren't overloaded with sodium. Or better yet, turn to fruits, vegetables, whole grains, and lean protein, which are naturally low in sodium and perfectly healthy for you and your baby.

Sodium-rich foods

Food	Portion	Sodium (mg)
Salt	1 teaspoon	2,300
Cheese pizza	1 slice	550
Fast-food chicken caesar salad	1 order	1,170
Soy sauce	1 tablespoon	1,030
Tomato juice	1 cup	875

vitamin A

Vitamin A, an important fat-soluble vitamin naturally found in green leafy vegetables, aids in vision, cell production for you and your baby, and immune system health. Furthering its importance for you, it also aids postpartum tissue repair. The daily requirement for adult women is 5,000 International Units (IU). However, this amount comes with a warning: Large doses of vitamin A (primarily from supplements providing 10,000 IU of vitamin K or higher) can cause birth defects and liver toxicity. But don't pass up on the kale or Brussels sprouts just yet; overdosing is nothing to worry about so long as your supplements are in check.

This fat-soluble vitamin can be found in both animal and plant foods in different forms. Retinal is a kind of pre-formed vitamin A that's found in animal products. Carotenoids are found in fruits and vegetables and get converted into vitamin A in the body. Milk products are also often fortified with vitamin A.

Vitamin K-rich foods

Sweet potato	Milk
Carrot	Liver
Spinach	Eggs
Kale	Fortified cereals
Brussels sprouts	Cheese

vitamin D

The daily recommended amount of 200 IUs of vitamin D doesn't increase during pregnancy, but that doesn't make it any less important! Its main role is to help your body absorb calcium from food and deposit it into your bones. It is also critical for the development of your baby's teeth and bones. The good news is, you can't get too much vitamin D. Your body either uses it immediately or stores it for later. Regular sun exposure would be enough of a source, except that many women do not get enough exposure to the sun or wear sunscreen, which prevents the process from starting. This is why it is important to find food sources of vitamin D. With the exception of a few foods, most of the vitamin D found in foods is fortified, and thus more available.

Natural sources of vitamin D	Fortified vitamin D
Mushrooms	Orange juice
Salmon	Milk
Sardines	Yogurt
Egg	Ready-to-eat cereal
Cheese	Margarine
Liver	

vitamin C

Vitamin C may be best known for its cold-fighting abilities, but it also helps in the production of collagen (which helps your now-stretching skin retain its elasticity), the formation and repair of red blood cells, and efficient iron absorption—all of which are especially helpful to you right now. Since it's water-soluble, it can't be stored in the body, which means that you need to reach your vitamin C requirements of 70 milligrams every day. Just one red bell pepper a day is actually enough to meet your vitamin C minimum.

Vitamin C–rich foods

Orange	Strawberries
Red bell pepper	Grapefruit
Kiwi	Lemon
Tomato	Lime

antioxidants

Antioxidants protect you and your baby's tissues from damage from free radicals (highly reactive oxygen fragments) and reduce the risk of damage to your baby's DNA. Additionally, studies have shown that healthy intakes of a specific antioxidant, vitamin E, during pregnancy can reduce your baby's risk of getting asthma down the road.

Spices such as cinnamon, oregano, parsley, basil, paprika, and ginger are all great sources of antioxidants, as are herbs like sage, peppermint, and tarragon, and foods such as dried fruits, nuts, and deeply pigmented fruits and vegetables.

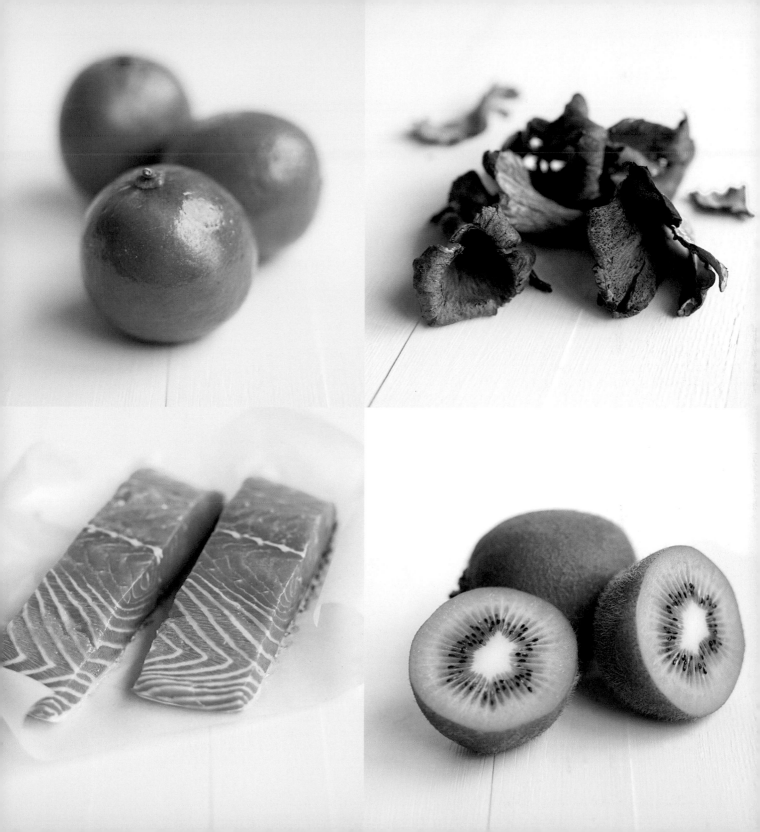

hydration

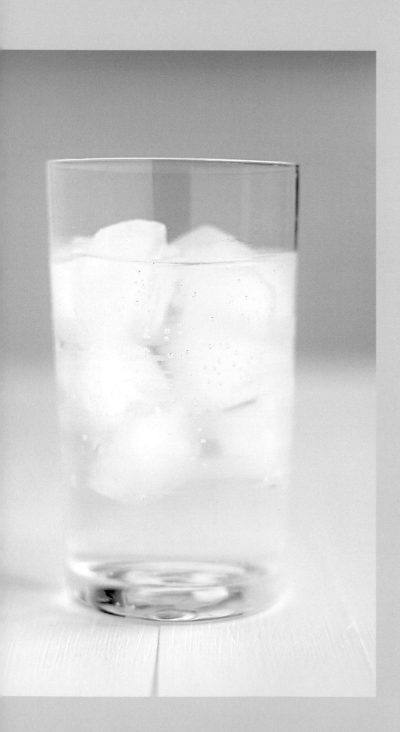

Staying hydrated is extremely important, even before pregnancy. Proper hydration allows your body to perform critical everyday functions, including regulating your body temperature, transporting and distributing nutrients to areas that need them, and helping to dispose of waste that, if stored in the body, can create illness.

When you're pregnant, drinking enough water is even more essential, as it ensures your body can properly cushion and protect your growing baby. It also aids in the production of your increased blood supply.

To make sure you are properly hydrated, drink at least 64 ounces (eight 8-ounce cups) of water or other hydrating fluids, such as milk, juice, or non-caffeinated teas, each day. Make sure you space them out throughout the day, and add a few extra glasses while you're at it. Your body will thank you for it.

Coffee, caffeinated tea, and soda do not count toward your total fluid intake because, as diuretics, they actually cause your body to lose water. Additionally, sugary sodas should be consumed sparingly, as they can increase your blood sugar and have no health benefits. Juice is a healthy choice, but it should be enjoyed in moderation since overindulgence in such high-calorie beverages can lead to excessive weight gain.

Drinking liquids isn't the only way to increase your fluid intake. Most produce contains ample amounts of water that aids in keeping you hydrated. That said, water from fruit and vegetables should be considered a bonus and should not replace the recommended number of glasses of water per day.

morning sickness

Any pregnant woman with this condition will tell you "morning sickness" is a misnomer. Nausea can be a constant and very unwelcome companion at any time of day or night, and studies show that up to 70 percent of women suffer from nausea, vomiting, or both sometime during pregnancy. For most women, the queasy feeling begins early in pregnancy, often as one of the first clues to her new condition, and tends to dissipate early in the second trimester—although it can last much longer, even straight through to delivery. No one is really sure why nausea occurs, but it's likely due to hormonal changes. There's no "best" way to quell morning sickness. Every woman reacts differently to the various popular solutions listed below. They are all worth trying.

1 Get up slowly in the morning and nibble on some plain crackers before getting out of bed.

2 Avoid nausea triggers. Certain smells or foods may be triggers for you, so avoid them as much as possible.

3 Eat snacks and light meals. Simple, plain foods like crackers can be really helpful when those nauseous waves first come on.

4 Eat small, frequent meals. An empty stomach can be extra-acidic, which can lead to extra heartburn or nausea. Overeating can also lead to discomfort.

5 Drink enough fluids. Dehydration can worsen your nausea; take small sips of water all day long to stay properly hydrated.

6 Avoid getting overheated. Heat can increase nausea symptoms.

7 Rest up! Nausea and fatigue often go hand in hand, so be sure to get enough sleep.

Call your health care provider if you experience uncontrolled vomiting, vomit two or more times daily, or can't keep any food or water down as you may be experiencing hyperemesis gravidarum and will need to be closely monitored by your doctor.

food aversions

Even if you don't experience morning sickness, you are likely to experience a time where certain foods that were once your friends have become your foes. Whether spicy foods now send you sprinting for the door or the sight of chicken makes your skin crawl, it's common to have some sort of food aversion at some point during pregnancy. Alas, no one knows what triggers these reactions, but at least they often disappear as quickly as they come on!

While there's no reason to force yourself to keep company with your temporary enemies, it is important to find an alternative source of the nutrients that food provides. If chicken is off the menu, consider beef or pork. If dairy products are hard to swallow, try getting calcium from plant-based foods, as discussed on page 17.

all-star food list

Getting all the nutrients you need is easier than you might think. Just make sure to have at least two of the following food groups in each meal and mix it up. That way you can be sure that you are getting all the important nutrients that you and your baby need.

★ Lean meat: protein, iron, vitamin B12

★ Fish: protein, calcium, healthy fat

★ Low-fat dairy: protein, calcium, vitamin A, riboflavin

★ Whole grains: folate, carbohydrates, fiber, iron

★ Fruits: fiber, antioxidants, carbohydrates, vitamin A, folate

★ Vegetables: fiber, antioxidants, vitamin A, calcium, iron

foods to avoid

For many pregnant women, eating is one of the highlights—and focuses—of pregnancy. Never before has food tasted so good or felt so imperative! But worrying if the food you are eating is safe or unsafe for your unborn baby can take the joy out of even the most vibrantly seasoned meal—especially because pregnancy-induced changes in your body's metabolism and circulation increase your risk of bacterial food poisoning, which can seriously affect your baby's well-being. To keep it simple—and safe—avoid the following list of "no-nos" and you can gorge worry-free!

no-no foods

Raw/undercooked or potentially contaminated seafood
Avoid raw fish and shellfish, heed local fish advisories (especially if you eat fish from local waters), cook seafood to an internal temperature of 145°F (63°C), and cook clams, mussels, and oysters until their shells open, discarding any that remain closed.

Undercooked meat, poultry, and eggs
Make sure meat and poultry is fully cooked before eating it; avoid hot dogs and processed deli meats, which can contain Listeria (a bacteria that can cause serious infection); and stay away from refrigerated patés and meat spreads. Instead, reach for canned and shelf-stable versions. Finally, be sure eggs are fully cooked to avoid the potential of contracting salmonella. That means thinking twice before licking the bowl of cookie or cake batter or ordering eggs Benedict or Caesar salad (often made with raw egg yolk) at a restaurant.

Seafood with high mercury content
Fish is a great source of protein and omega-3 fatty acids and should be part of a healthy pregnancy diet. But certain fish have potentially dangerous levels of a metal called mercury that could damage your unborn baby's nervous system. If you're not sure which fish is safe, a quick tip is to avoid bigger fish as they contain more mercury. Even fish considered "safe" should be eaten in moderation, or up to 12 ounces (340 grams) a week.

Fish to avoid

Swordfish
Shark
King mackerel
Tilefish

Fish to eat in moderation

Shrimp
Canned light tuna (but limit albacore tuna and tuna steak to once per week)
Salmon
Pollock
Catfish
Cod

Unpasteurized foods
Avoid foods, such as cheese, milk and juices, that have not been "pasteurized" (sterilized through heating), as they may carry bacteria that can cause foodborne illnesses.

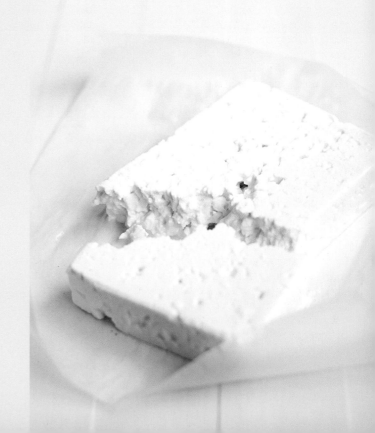

Unless their packaging clearly states that the following cheeses are pasteurized, avoid them:
Brie
Feta
Camembert
Blue cheese
Mexican-style cheeses (queso blanco, queso fresco, and panela)

Large quantities of liver
Avoid overindulging in this offal meat, as it is a significant source of vitamin A and can be dangerous to your baby if consumed in large amounts.

Unwashed fruits and vegetables
Wash your fruits and vegetables prior to eating them to avoid potential exposure to toxoplasmosis, an infection due to parasites found in some soils.

Excess caffeine
Take it easy on coffee, tea, and other caffeinated beverages, as they can cross the placenta and their effects on your baby are still not fully known. If you can't bear the thought of going a day without a caffeine boost, keep your intake to less than 300 (milligrams) mg of caffeine per day. (To put that in perspective, a typical 8-ounce cup of coffee has 100 mg of caffeine, decaffeinated only has 3 mg, and 8 ounces of brewed tea has approximately 40 to 60 mg of caffeine.) Caffeine is also a diuretic and can cause water and calcium loss.

Alcohol
While guidelines differ slightly throughout the world, the safest bet is to avoid alcohol during your pregnancy, especially because there is really no amount of alcohol that has been proven safe to drink. If you indulged with abandon before you knew you were pregnant, it's not worth stressing over. There's nothing you can do about it now, and plenty of women before you have done the same and gone on to have healthy children. Still, it's a proven fact that excessive alcohol consumption during pregnancy can lead to fetal alcohol syndrome, which encompasses a collection of mental and physical problems in your baby, as well as other developmental disorders, so why not hold off until you can toast your new family?

Of all the possible pregnancy-related discomforts, several of them can be influenced—for better and for worse—by what you eat. Besides morning sickness, the following are three of the most common food-related irritants, along with tips on how to relieve them.

Constipation
Pregnancy slows down the movement of food through your digestive tract and can cause constipation, as can the iron supplements you're taking. But fiber can help. Increase your fresh fruit and vegetable intake for an increase in fiber. Also add dried fruit to your diet and aim for at least six to eight glasses of water a day.

Diarrhea
Diarrhea is sometimes caused by hormonal changes, lactose intolerance, or sensitivities to certain foods while pregnant. To combat it, eat more foods that help absorb excess water. Bananas, rice, applesauce, and bread are the four all-stars for watery bowel movements. Also, be sure to drink a lot of water to replace the lost fluids.

Heartburn
Heartburn is common in the beginning of pregnancy due to the hormonal changes that slow down your digestive system. Later, as the baby grows, there is crowding near your stomach, which causes stomach acid to back up into the esophagus. To avoid it, eat small, frequent meals throughout the day; try drinking milk before eating; and limit caffeinated foods and beverages.

Water retention
Those hormones again—or too much salt in your diet—can cause water retention. To quell it, increase your water intake and put your feet up. Eat plenty of water-rich foods like fresh fruits and vegetables. See your doctor if the swelling increases rapidly or causes any discomfort because such symptoms can be associated with preeclampsia.

vegetarian tips

Vegetarianism can be an extremely healthy lifestyle for pregnant women, especially because studies show vegetarians are more likely to consume whole grains, legumes, and vegetables than meat eaters. Additionally, since vegetarians can get protein and other nutrients from dairy products, eggs, or both, daily dietary requirements tend to be very easy to come by. Vegans, however, need to be more diligent about getting all the important nutrients usually associated with meat and dairy—especially protein, iron, calcium, vitamins D and B12, zinc, and folate—during pregnancy.

So whether you've been a vegan or vegetarian for years, have suddenly lost that loving feeling for meat and fish, or want to remain carnivorous but also reap some of the health benefits from a vegetarian diet, you should turn to the following alternatives for getting the important nutrients found in animal products.

protein

If you are a lacto-ovo vegetarian (meaning you eat dairy and eggs), finding protein sources is pretty easy. Just load up on eggs, milk, and yogurt. For vegans, meeting daily nutritional needs is more of a challenge, but can be done by consuming a wide variety of plant-based foods, such as whole grains, legumes, soy, and vegetables. For information on the importance of protein during pregnancy, see page 14.

Protein sources

Soy products (soy milk, tofu, tempeh)
Beans and legumes
Nuts/nut butters
Whole grains (especially quinoa)

iron

Iron requirements increase so much when you're pregnant that even meat-eaters have a hard time meeting their iron needs. Most prenatal vitamins contain iron, however, it's also important to eat iron from healthy, natural sources—and pair iron-rich foods with vitamin C to increase absorption. For more on iron and pregnancy, see page 18.

Iron sources

Chickpeas
Dried fruit
Lentils

calcium

You need calcium to help your baby grow strong bones, teeth, muscles and nerves, and a healthy heart. Dairy products are great sources of this bone-building nutrient, as are calcium-rich plant foods like tofu, broccoli, okra, and oranges. See more about calcium on page 17.

vitamin D

Vitamin D aids in the absorption of calcium, but few foods naturally contain it. Still, it is easily found in fortified milk products and ready-to-eat cereals. For vegans, fortified soy milk is a good source, but it's still worth asking your health care provider if you should take a supplement.

B12

Out of all the B vitamins, B12 is the biggest concern for vegetarians and vegans, since it is mainly found in animal products. Pregnant women who avoid meat need to make a concerted effort to eat plant-based food sources of vitamin B12, such as fortified soy milk, to prevent anemia. A fortified breakfast cereal with milk or fortified soy milk is a great and healthy way to get your B12.

good go-to snacks

During pregnancy, eating enough to keep your blood sugar stable as well as meeting the nutritional needs of you and your growing baby is often a challenge. Go too long and your body will certainly let you know; as you can probably attest, there is no desperation like that of a hungry pregnant woman. That's why it's a good idea to keep snacks on hand at all times. Stick a few in your purse or lunch bag and you'll be able to tame your tummy before it starts to roar.

1 Low-fat yogurt
2 Apple with nut butter
3 Peanut Butter Chocolate Chip Energy Bars (see page 47)
4 Sesame-Honey Almonds (see page 47)
5 String cheese
6 Hummus and Crudités (see page 51)
7 Fruit Salad with Orange-Ginger Syrup (see page 52)
8 Fortified ready-to-eat cereal
9 Glass of skim milk or soy milk
10 Edamame or roasted soybeans

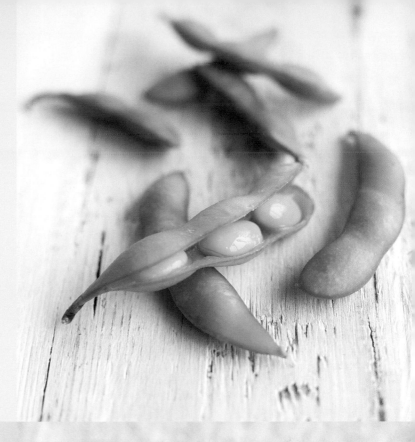

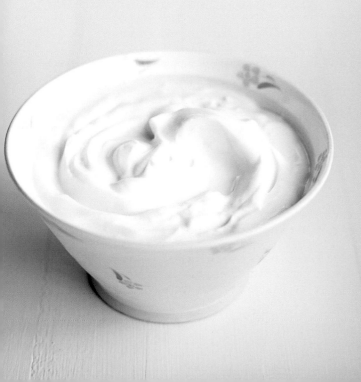

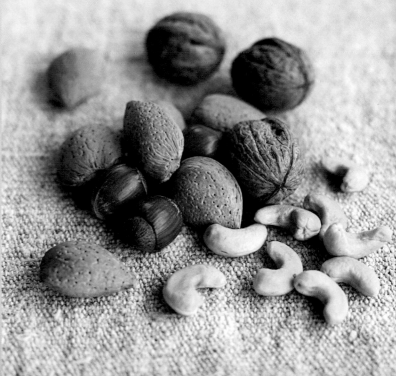

sleep

The art of sleep becomes a whole new skill when you are pregnant. During the first trimester, you may have a hard time keeping your eyes open or you may suffer from bouts of insomnia. In your second and third trimesters, back pain, heartburn, or the sheer awkwardness of your protruding belly may make it hard to sleep soundly. The fact is, your body is going through a multitude of changes in its growth and hormones, and these tend to disrupt sleep. Ironically, getting enough sleep is important for you and your baby. Here are some things you can try to improve slumber.

1   Avoid drinking anything at least an hour before bed, but be sure to stay well hydrated during the day.

2   Avoid eating anything at least an hour before bed to prevent heartburn from keeping you awake.

3   Avoid exercising in the evening, unless it's a relaxing walk or a yoga or meditation class.

4   Turn off all electronics well before bedtime, allow yourself to fully shut off.

5   Try drinking Warm Vanilla Milk (page 138) or have a cup of herbal tea.

exercise

If you don't have a high-risk pregnancy, exercise is extremely beneficial to both you and your baby. Proper exercise can help keep your weight gain under control and can lessen common pregnancy complaints such as sore legs and stiffness. Exercise can also boost your energy level and may even shorten labor and recovery time. It's important to remember that pregnancy is not the time to try to lose weight or achieve any major fitness goal, such as running a marathon.

However, exercising even just three to four days per week for at least 20 to 30 minutes will have tremendous health benefits for you and baby. Here are some important exercise guidelines to follow to keep you and baby safe and healthy.

1   Lower your intensity level; with your increased blood volume you really are working out for two!

2   Make sure you are well hydrated and have consumed enough calories before and after you exercise.

3   Don't do deep stretching or jerky, bouncy motions. Your body will tell you what not to do, so listen to it!

4   Don't allow yourself to get overheated

5   Do resume your workouts gradually after giving birth when your health care provider gives you the go-ahead.

let's get cooking

Now that you know what your body needs and why, here's the fun part: You can easily nourish yourself and your baby by whipping up the outstanding dishes in the following pages. Because there is no "perfect" diet for the pregnant woman, all you need to do is to cook and savor a wide variety of the recipes. Even better is that each one was created with the busy mom-to-be in mind, which means they are made from readily available ingredients and easy and quick to prepare.

That said, there are a few important things to keep in mind as you stock your kitchen. First and foremost is to buy organic fruits and vegetables whenever you can. Pesticides aren't good for you, your baby, or anyone else for that matter, and they can be found in pretty much everything that isn't organically grown. Yes, organic foods are expensive, but if you can afford it, it's money well spent. At a minimum, splurge on organic celery; peaches; strawberries; apples; blueberries; nectarines; sweet bell peppers; spinach, kale, and collard greens; cherries; potatoes; grapes; and lettuce—all of which have enough residual pesticides to be termed "the dirty dozen" by healthy-food advocacy groups.

Now, I know you've got the appetite, so please bite into the following recipes unabashedly! If you're like me, you will find they are tasty and practical enough to return to once you have a larger family to feed, especially because many of them are kid-friendly and so easy to prepare that you can practically whip them up with a baby hanging off your hip.

pantry essentials

Make life easy on yourself and stock up on pantry essentials that you can regularly reach for when cooking from this book:

- olive oil
- canola oil
- champagne vinegar
- rice vinegar
- sherry wine vinegar
- cartons of chicken or vegetable stock
- low-sodium soy sauce
- old-fashioned rolled oats
- sliced almonds
- maple syrup
- honey
- vanilla
- kosher salt
- black peppercorns
- dijon mustard
- garlic
- fresh ginger
- pasteurized feta

It wouldn't hurt to add some organic berries and carrots, eggs, plain non-fat Greek yogurt, and frozen shrimp to your shopping basket, since they are great last-minute, go-to ingredients or easily prepared mini meals, even if you're not cooking from this book.

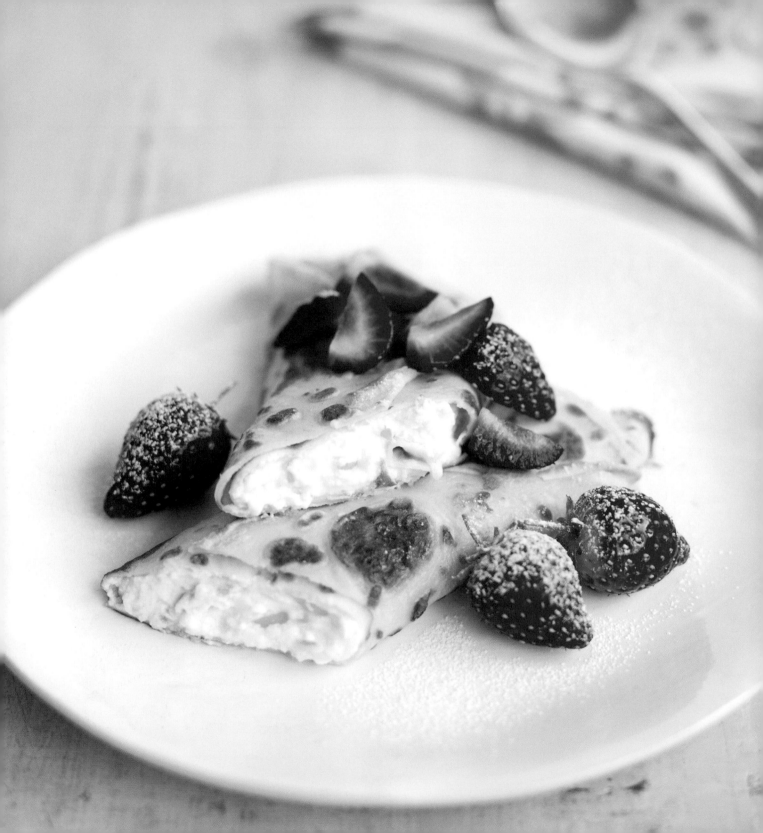

chapter one
breakfast foods

nutrient-rich granola

The great thing about granola is that it's easy to make in bulk and even easier to customize. Plus, it can serve as a wholesome, energy-rich breakfast or snack when paired with milk or sprinkled over yogurt or cottage cheese. This particular mixture ups the health factor with omega-3-rich pumpkin seeds, protein-packed peanuts, and oats, which are full of dietary fiber. Feel free to add other nuts, dried fruit, or both!

Serves 16

3 cups rolled oats
½ cup pumpkin seeds
½ cup slivered almonds
¼ cup dark brown sugar
3 tablespoons honey

¼ cup vegetable oil
1½ teaspoons ground cardamom
½ teaspoon kosher salt
½ cup raisins

Preheat the oven to 250°F.

In a large bowl, combine the oats, pumpkin seeds, almond slivers, and brown sugar.

In another bowl, combine the honey, oil, cardamom, and salt. Combine both mixtures and spread evenly on one large, or two smaller, baking sheets. Bake for 1 hour and 15 minutes, stirring every 15 minutes for even color.

Remove from the oven, cool, and transfer to a sealable container. Add the raisins and mix until evenly distributed. Store, covered, to maintain freshness.

PER SERVING: 176 CALORIES, 8.62G FAT, 1.09G CARBS, 5.28G PROTEIN, 2.33G FIBER, 23MG CALCIUM, 2.03MG IRON, 75MG SODIUM, 10µG FOLATE

yogurt, granola, and strawberry parfait

An ideal way to start a morning or satisfy midday hunger pangs, this melange of fruit, yogurt, and granola looks beautiful when layered in a dessert glass, but tastes just as good served in a bowl. And it provides protein, dietary fiber, vitamin C, folate, and potassium.

Serves 1

¼ cup granola (store-bought or see recipe on this page)
¾ cup plain Greek yogurt
1 teaspoon honey
¾ cup strawberries, quartered
sprig mint, for garnish

Place the granola in a glass or bowl. Top with the yogurt. Drizzle with the honey and finish with a layer of strawberries and a mint garnish. Bon appétit!

PER SERVING: 311 CALORIES, 7.53G FAT, 45.73G CARBS, 15.91G PROTEIN, FIBER, 407MG CALCIUM, 2.00MG IRON, 149MG SODIUM, 76µG FOLATE

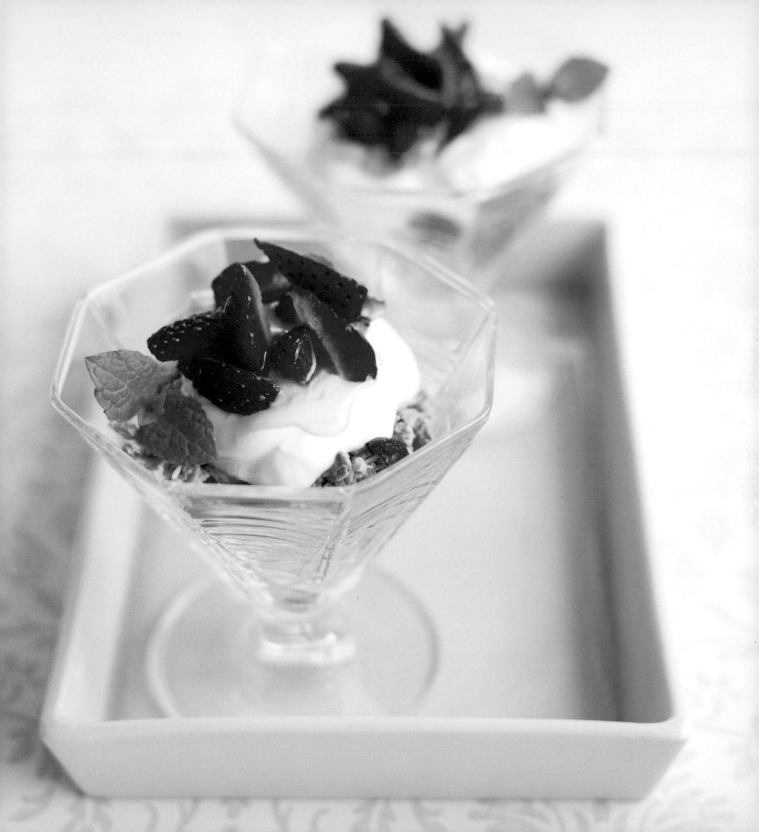

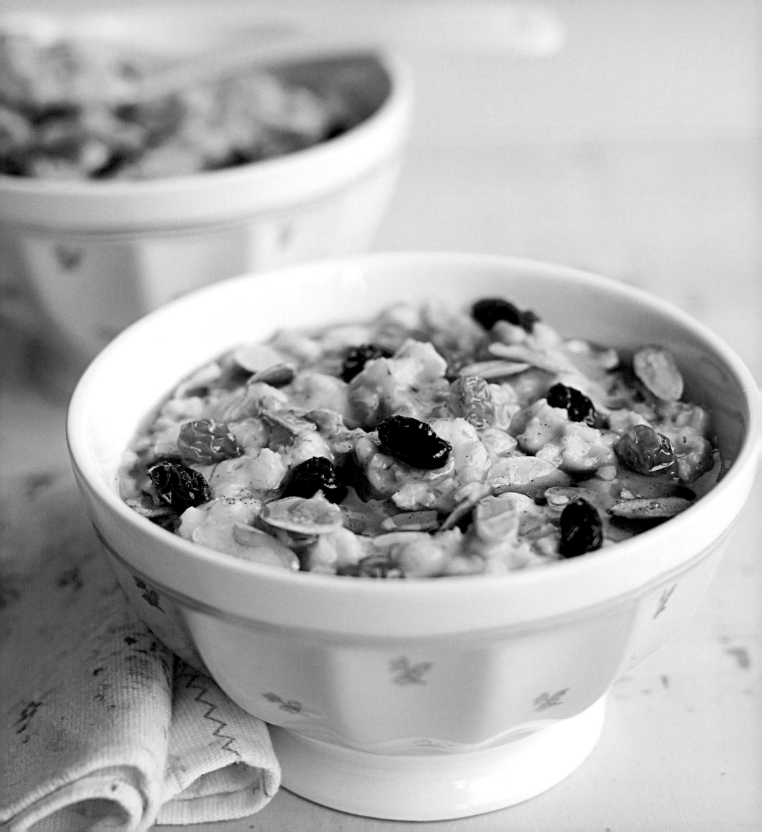

maple oatmeal with raisins and almonds

Wonderfully filling and containing heart-healthy fiber and antioxidants, oatmeal is also an excellent source of manganese, a mineral that helps you and your baby form bone and cartilage.

Serves 1

½ cup water
½ cup low-fat milk
¼ teaspoon kosher salt
½ cup rolled oats
½ teaspoon vanilla extract
1 tablespoon raisins
2 teaspoons toasted sliced almonds
1 tablespoon pure maple syrup

In a small saucepan, bring the water, milk, and salt to a boil. Add the oats and vanilla, reduce the heat to low, and cook for 10 to 20 minutes, stirring occasionally, until it's your desired consistency. Add additional water if necessary.

Transfer the oatmeal to a serving bowl and top with the raisins and almonds. Drizzle with the maple syrup.

PER SERVING: 328 CALORIES, 5.39G FAT, 59.67G CARBS, 11.56G PROTEIN, 4.75G FIBER, 225MG CALCIUM, 2.58MG IRON, 659MG SODIUM, 20µG FOLATE

asparagus, gruyère, and shallot scramble

The decadence of rich cheese, sweet caramelized shallots, and fresh asparagus should be enough reason to break out your frying pan to whip up this quick breakfast, which is my mom's recipe. But here's an even better excuse: Asparagus imparts excellent amounts of folate—which is essential for a baby's development, especially early in pregnancy—and eggs and cheese are wonderful protein sources.

Serves 4

2 teaspoons canola oil
2 teaspoons unsalted butter
½ cup minced shallots
20 asparagus stalks (green part only),
    sliced at an angle into ⅓-inch pieces
8 eggs
4 teaspoons water
½ teaspoon kosher salt
1 pinch freshly ground black pepper
1 cup loosely packed grated Gruyère
    (approximately 6 ounces)

Heat the oil and butter in a large nonstick sauté pan over medium heat. Add the shallots and asparagus and cook until the asparagus is cooked but still somewhat crisp and the shallots have not yet browned.

In a bowl, mix the eggs, water, salt, and pepper thoroughly, then add to the pan. Sprinkle the grated cheese on top of the egg mixture and gently stir until the eggs are fully cooked. Serve.

PER SERVING: 294 CALORIES, 18.42G FAT, 5.65G CARBS, 22.66G PROTEIN, 1.68G FIBER, 348 MG CALCIUM, 3.71MG IRON, 233MG SODIUM, 94µG FOLATE

portobello and black bean breakfast burritos

Robustly flavored by meaty portobello mushrooms, this vegetarian meal can be prepared in advance. Refrigerate or freeze a couple of burritos for a quick protein-rich meal later.

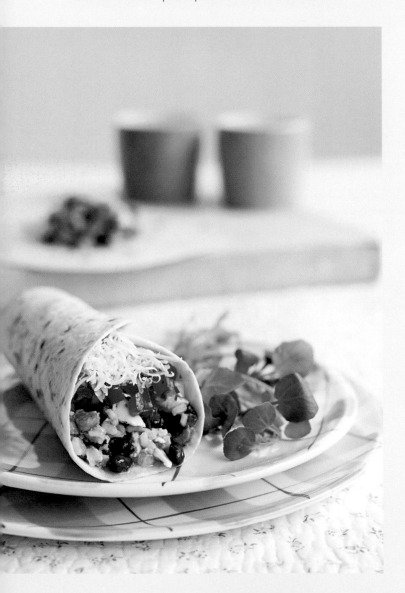

Serves 4

4 large flour tortillas
1 tablespoon plus 1 teaspoon olive oil
1 cup diced onion (from 1 small onion)
1 tablespoon minced fresh garlic
2 large portobello mushrooms, diced
3 tablespoons lemon juice
1 tablespoon brown rice miso paste
1 tablespoon hoisin sauce
½ teaspoon kosher salt
1 dash Tabasco (or more to taste)
1 cup canned black beans, rinsed and drained
1 cup cooked brown rice
4 egg whites
½ cup grated Monterey Jack cheese (optional)
½ cup salsa (optional)

Preheat the oven to 350°F. Wrap the tortillas tightly in a large sheet of foil and warm in oven until heated through, 10 to 15 minutes. Keep warm.

Meanwhile, heat the oil in a large sauté pan until hot but not smoking. Cook the onion, garlic, and mushrooms, stirring occasionally, until browned, 8 to 10 minutes.

In a small bowl, whisk together the lemon juice, miso paste, hoisin sauce, salt, and Tabasco. Pour over the mushrooms. Transfer to a food processor and pulse until well chopped but not pulverized. Return to the pan and add the black beans, brown rice, and egg whites and cook over medium heat, stirring, until the egg whites are fully cooked.

Place a warm tortilla on a plate. Spoon ¼ of the mushroom mixture, ¼ of the cheese, and ¼ of the salsa, if using, in vertical rows across the center, leaving room on the bottom and sides of the tortilla. Fold the bottom over most of the filling, then fold over the sides, overlapping them. Repeat with the other 3 burritos. Serve hot.

PER SERVING: 642 CALORIES, 12.52G FAT, 84.48G CARBS, 7.50G FIBER, 21.60G PROTEIN, 255MG CALCIUM, 4.10MG IRON, 1125MG SODIUM, 101µG FOLATE

zucchini, basil, and parmesan frittata

This vegetarian dish is a basil and roasted bell pepper riff on famed New York chef Eric Ripert's Zucchini Mint Parmesan Frittata. It does double duty as a healthful way to start the day or a perfect luncheon partner, especially if paired with a small green salad.

Serves 6

8 large eggs
2 zucchini, julienned (about 1¾ cups)
1 roasted red bell pepper, julienned
¼ cup freshly grated Parmesan
20 basil leaves, torn into pieces
½ teaspoon kosher salt
freshly ground black pepper
1½ teaspoons olive oil

Preheat the oven to 325°F.

In a stainless-steel bowl, whisk the eggs well. Add the zucchini, roasted red pepper, Parmesan, basil, salt, and pepper and stir to combine.

Heat the olive oil in a 9- or 10-inch ovenproof skillet over medium heat, swirling the oil to coat the bottom and sides. Pour in the egg mixture and cook, without stirring, for 3 minutes, or until it begins to pull away from the skillet.

Transfer the skillet to the oven and bake for 12 to 15 minutes, or until the eggs are set and firm in the center.

Remove from the oven and gently run a rubber spatula around the sides of the skillet to loosen the frittata. For an elegant presentation, place a serving plate over the skillet and carefully flip the pan to invert the frittata onto the serving plate. Cut into wedges and serve warm or at room temperature. Or simply serve straight from the skillet.

PER SERVING: 164 CALORIES, 8.05G FAT, 6.14G CARBS, 13.23G PROTEIN, 2.42G FIBER, 232MG CALCIUM, 4.11MG IRON, 163MG SODIUM, 113µG FOLATE

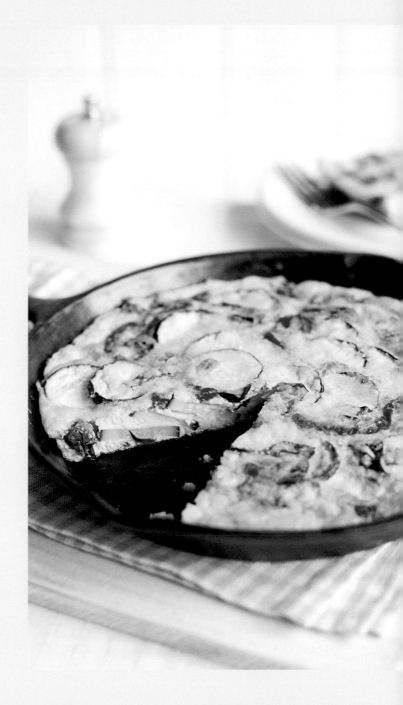

cottage cheese pancake and strawberry "omelets"

A denser, more nutritious answer to a breakfast favorite, these extra-moist pancakes are served folded like omelets, stuffed with sliced strawberries, drizzled with maple syrup, and sprinkled with powdered sugar—all of which makes them look and taste like dessert! Be sure to use organic strawberries, which include all the fruit's nutrients without the pesticides found in non-organic options. Also, feel free to up the health factor by using whole-wheat flour.

Serves 4

$2/3$ cup low-fat cottage cheese
1 cup whole-wheat flour
2 large eggs
4 egg whites
2 tablespoons honey
2 tablespoons low-fat milk
1 teaspoon vanilla extract
¼ teaspoon ground cinnamon
pinch of kosher salt
1 teaspoon canola oil
2 cups organic strawberries, sliced
4 teaspoons maple syrup
2 teaspoons powdered sugar
4 sprigs mint (optional)

Preheat the oven to 200°F. In a large bowl, mix the cottage cheese, flour, eggs, egg whites, honey, milk, vanilla, cinnamon, and salt.

Heat the oil in a large nonstick skillet over medium heat, swirling the oil to coat the bottom of the skillet. Pour ¼ of the batter onto the skillet, tilting so the batter spreads as evenly and thinly to coat the bottom. Cook until the bottom is brown and bubbles form on top, about 3 minutes. Flip and cook until the other side is brown and the pancake is cooked through, about 3 minutes. Transfer to a plate and keep warm in the oven. Repeat with the remaining batter until there are 4 pancakes.

When all the pancakes are cooked, transfer each to a plate, top with ½ cup of sliced strawberries, and drizzle with 1 teaspoon maple syrup. Fold the pancake in half so it's shaped like an omelet. Sprinkle with powdered sugar, garnish with a mint sprig, if using. Repeat with the remaining "omelets" and serve.

PER SERVING: 282 CALORIES, 4.41G FAT, 45.16G CARBS, 5.52G FIBER, 16.25G PROTEIN, 92MG CALCIUM, 2.37MG IRON, 294MG SODIUM, 51µG FOLATE

totally tasty breakfast muffins

Taking the lead from award-winning cookbook author James Peterson's carrot cake recipe, this recipe makes impossibly moist, dessert-like muffins that are loaded with vegetables, good fats (from the nuts and seeds)—which are essential for a developing baby brain—and even fresh fruit. Munch on them for a week or freeze a batch for future late-night snack attacks. They're a great way to get vegetables, fiber, and antioxidants without even trying!

Makes 12 muffins

2 teaspoons butter
2/3 cup flour plus more for flouring the pan
1/3 cup sugar
1 teaspoon baking soda
3/4 teaspoon baking powder
1 teaspoon ground cinnamon
1/4 teaspoon nutmeg
1/4 teaspoon ground allspice
1/4 teaspoon kosher salt
1/3 cup vegetable oil
2 eggs
1/3 cup pumpkin seeds (optional)
1 cup chopped walnuts
2/3 cup finely grated zucchini
1/2 cup peeled and finely grated sweet
   red apple
1 cup finely grated carrot

Preheat the oven to 350°F. Butter and flour the muffin pan if it is not nonstick.

In a bowl, sift together the 2/3 cup flour, the sugar, baking soda, baking powder, cinnamon, nutmeg, allspice, and salt, and mix to combine.

In a small bowl, whisk together the oil and eggs until blended, and then stir the egg mixture into the flour.

In a coffee grinder or food processor, grind the pumpkin seeds into a coarse meal. Mix into the batter, along with the walnuts, zucchini, apple, and carrot.

Divide the batter evenly among the 12 muffin cups and bake for 15 to 18 minutes, or until a toothpick inserted in the center comes out clean. Cool on a wire rack, then run a knife around the edges of each muffin and gently remove from the pan. Serve warm or at room temperature.

PER SERVING: 220 CALORIES, 15.93G FAT, 15.09G CARBS, 1.59G FIBER, 5.36G PROTEIN, 41MG CALCIUM, 1.82MG IRON, 202MG SODIUM, 31µG FOLATE

ricotta-cheese blintzes with blueberry sauce

Let's be honest: These dessert-like treats are not exactly pillars of healthy eating. However, of all the sweet, syrup-laden breakfasts out there, these provide protein from the ricotta as well as vitamin C, dietary fiber, and antioxidants from the blueberries. They are also look pretty enough to be special-occasion fare. Want to make them more guilt-free? Use the ripest, sweetest blueberries you can find, and cut back on the amount of sugar. Or skip the blueberries altogether and top with sliced fresh strawberries.

Serves 4

2 eggs
¼ cup skim milk
⅓ cup water
1 tablespoon vegetable oil
⅔ cup all-purpose flour
¼ teaspoon plus 2 tablespoons sugar
pinch of kosher salt
1 cup ricotta cheese
⅓ cup powdered sugar
½ teaspoon finely grated zest
2 tablespoons fresh lemon juice
1 cup fresh organic blueberries
¾ teaspoons cornstarch

In a large bowl, whisk together 1 egg and the milk, water, and oil. Whisk in the flour, ¼ teaspoon sugar, and salt until smooth.

Heat a medium nonstick skillet over medium-high heat. Ladle ¼ of the batter onto the skillet, tilting so the batter evenly coats the bottom. Cook until light brown on both sides, turning once, 2 to 4 minutes. Transfer to a platter and repeat with the remaining batter, separating the crepes with small squares of wax paper.

Preheat the oven to 350° F. Butter a 9 x 13-inch baking dish or spray it with cooking spray.

In a bowl, beat the remaining egg and stir in the ricotta, powdered sugar, lemon zest, and 1 tablespoon lemon juice. Spoon about 2 tablespoons of the cheese mixture on a crepe; fold up the top and bottom like a letter, tucking the ends in to keep the filling from leaking. Repeat with the remaining ingredients until there are 4 blintzes. Arrange the filled blintzes in the baking dish and bake for 20 minutes.

In a pot, combine the blueberries, remaining 1 tablespoon lemon juice, 2 tablespoons sugar, and cornstarch and cook over medium heat, stirring frequently until the berries burst, about 5 minutes. Remove from the heat and keep warm.

To serve, place one blintz on a plate and top with ¼ of the berry mixture.

PER SERVING: 346 CALORIES, 13.37G FAT, 43.10G CARBS, 2.12G FIBER, 13.21G PROTEIN, 185MG CALCIUM, 1.15MG IRON, 168MG SODIUM, 27µG FOLATE

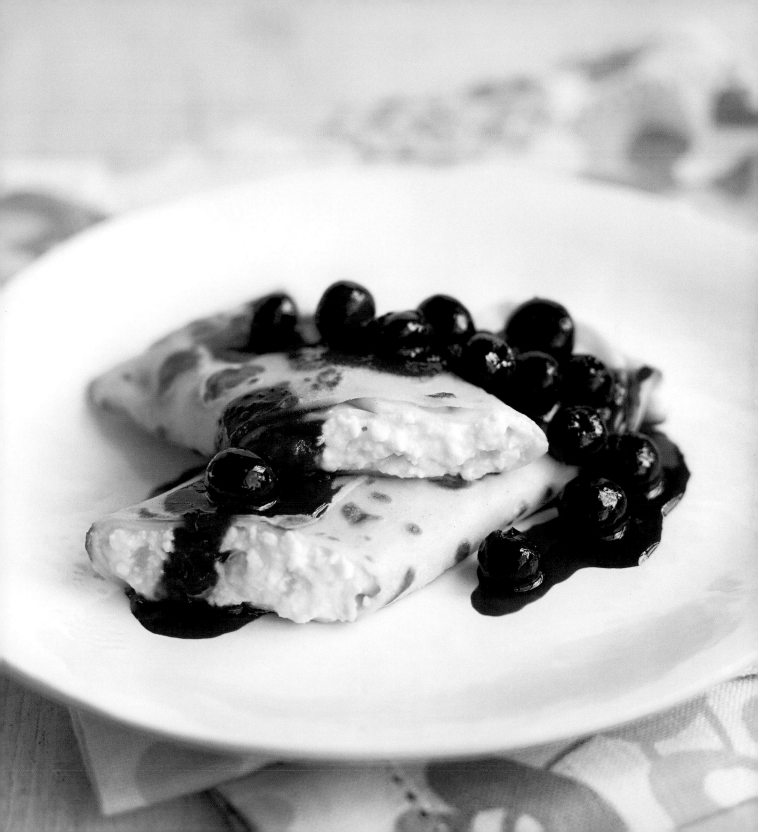

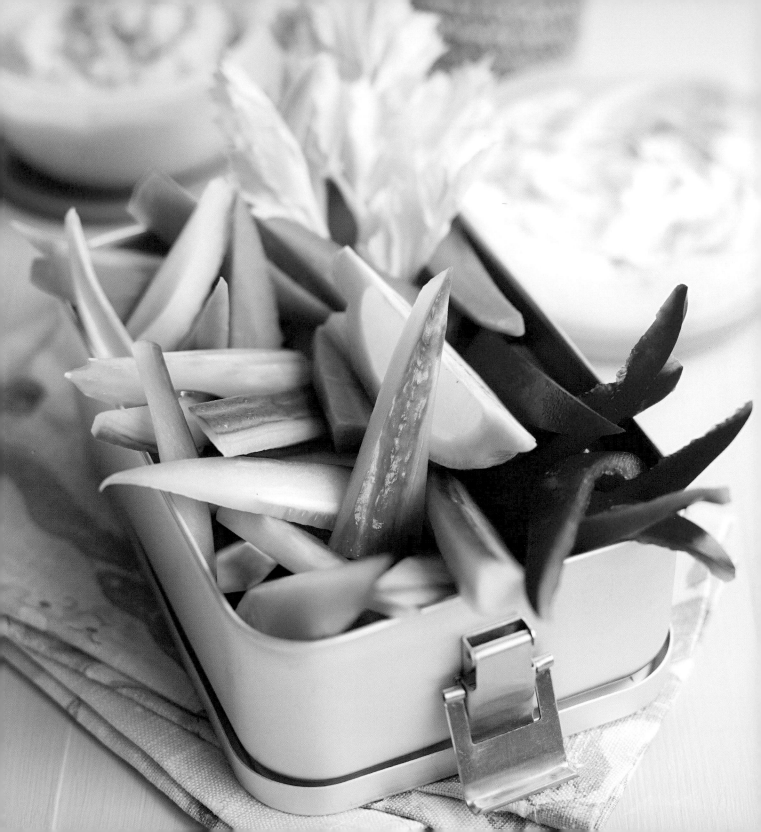

chapter two
snacks

roasted carrot chews

parmesan-dusted kale chips

When easy-to-grab snacks are essential to everyday sanity, it's a good idea to have healthy options on hand. These rustic, chewy, sweet, and salty carrot bites rise to the appetite-curbing occasion, and they taste great, too. Even better: carrots are brimming with good stuff, including vitamins A, C, K, and B6, potassium, and fiber. Want to fancy them up? Sprinkle them with a tablespoon of minced parsley leaves.

No need to force yourself to eat dark leafy greens with this genius recipe from *The Real Deal Guide to Pregnancy*'s Web site, realdealguide.com. The crisp texture and delicious flavor of these "chips" garner almost the same adoration as the less-nutritional potato-based bites. But unlike their greasier competition, they're super-low in calories and loaded with vitamins A, C, and K, a better source of calcium than spinach!

Serves 4

10 large carrots, unpeeled
2 teaspoons olive oil
1 teaspoon kosher salt

Serves 4

1 bunch of fresh green kale
1 tablespoon olive oil
¼ cup freshly grated Parmesan

Preheat the oven to 400ºF.

Slice the carrots diagonally in ½-inch-thick slices. Toss them in a bowl with the olive oil and salt until they are evenly coated. Spread the carrots on a baking sheet in one layer and roast for 30 minutes.

Let the carrots cool, season with additional salt, if desired, and snack in good conscience.

Preheat the oven to 250ºF.

Cut out the center stems of the kale leaves and discard. Slice each kale leaf into 4-inch strips. Toss them in a bowl with the olive oil, then evenly sprinkle with the cheese. Spread the kale on a baking sheet in a single layer and bake for 30 minutes or until crisp.

Cool and serve unabashedly.

PER SERVING: 93 CALORIES, 2.49G FAT, 17.24G CARBS, 1.67G PROTEIN, 5.04G FIBER, 59 MG CALCIUM, 0.56MG IRON, 705MG SODIUM, 34µG FOLATE

PER SERVING: 90 CALORIES, 5.28G FAT, 6.96G CARBS, 4.61G PROTEIN, 1.34G FIBER, 159MG CALCIUM, 1.21MG IRON, 124MG SODIUM, 19µG FOLATE

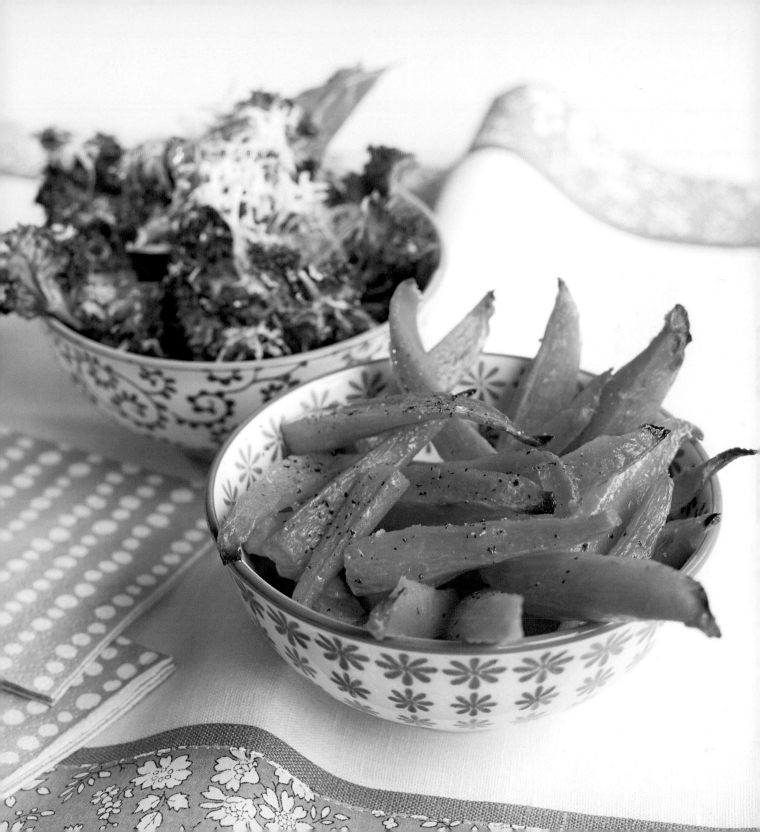

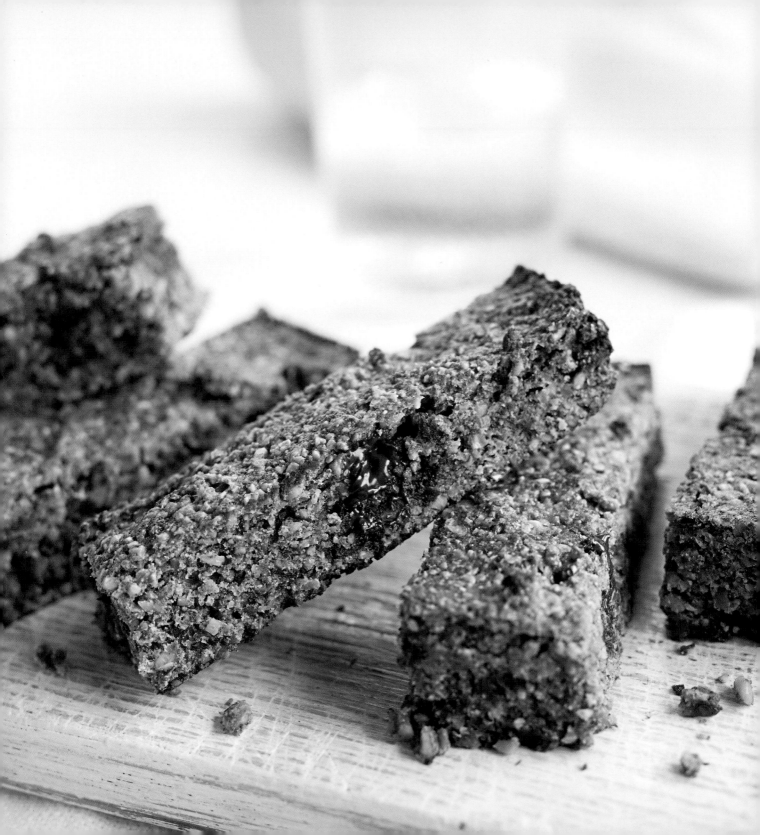

peanut butter chocolate chip energy bars

You can't beat snacks that are freshly made with wholesome ingredients. Modestly sweet with a flavor boost of salt, these peanut butter bites are full of protein and folate.

Makes 20 bars

½ teaspoon vegetable oil
1 cup quick-cooking rolled oats
1 cup dry-roasted peanuts
½ cup peanut butter
½ cup sunflower seeds
20 Medjool dates, pitted
2 eggs
1 teaspoon kosher salt
1 teaspoon vanilla
½ cup chocolate chips

Preheat the oven to 350°F. Lightly grease a 9 x 9-inch baking pan with vegetable oil and line the bottom with parchment paper.

Put the oats, peanuts, peanut butter, sunflower seeds, and dates in a food processor and pulse until finely chopped.

In a bowl, whisk the eggs together with the salt and vanilla, then add to the food processor, and pulse until the mixture becomes a coarse, chunky paste. Fold in the chocolate chips with a wooden spoon. Transfer the mixture to the prepared baking pan and spread evenly, gently pressing down to flatten. Bake for 35 minutes or until firm and golden.

Cool and cut into 20 bars. Store in an airtight container for a week in the refrigerator and a month in the freezer.

PER BAR: 164 CALORIES, 10.31G FAT, 14.51G CARBS, 5.39G PROTEIN, 2.57G FIBER, 16MG CALCIUM, 1.00MG IRON, 153MG SODIUM, 28µG FOLATE

sesame-honey almonds

A fantastic on-the-go snack and treat all in one, these protein- and calcium-loaded almonds are best made in bulk so you can grab a handful whenever you want. The only challenge is not to eat them all in one sitting.

Serves 16

3 cups sesame seeds
½ teaspoon coarse salt
5 tablespoons honey
2 tablespoons sugar
3 cups almonds

Preheat the oven to 350°F.

Place the sesame seeds in a large bowl and sprinkle the salt evenly over them.

In a pot, heat the honey and sugar over medium heat, stirring, until the mixture is runny. Working in batches, add the almonds to the hot mixture, stir to coat, quickly remove with a slotted spoon—letting the extra liquid drain off—and transfer the nuts to the bowl of sesame seeds.

Stir to coat with the sesame seeds, then transfer the nuts to a parchment paper-lined baking sheet.

Repeat until all the nuts are coated. Bake the sesame-coated almonds for 10 to 12 minutes.

Cool completely and store in an airtight container with a tight-sealing lid.

PER SERVING: 316 CALORIES, 23.49G FAT, 18.94G CARBS, 9.77G PROTEIN, 6.63G FIBER, 307MG CALCIUM, 4.56MG IRON, 75M SODIUM, 36µG FOLATE

japanese-style cold tofu

If you need a quick protein fix and your palate is craving pure, clean flavors, try this traditional Japanese dish. Called *hiyayakko*, it's elegant, easy to prepare, and refreshingly cold—making it perfect for cooling the engine and appetite of the overheating mother-to-be. Don't sweat it if you don't have access to bonito flakes. While they add interesting texture and a hint of fish flavor, the dish will satisfy without them.

Serves 4

4 (3-ounce) pieces of soft silken tofu
4 teaspoons chopped green onion
1 teaspoon grated fresh ginger
8 teaspoons dried bonito flakes (*katsuobushi*)
4 teaspoons soy sauce

Place the tofu in four individual bowls. Top each piece with 1 teaspoon green onion, ¼ teaspoon grated ginger, and 2 teaspoons bonito flakes.

Pour 1 teaspoon soy sauce over each tofu and enjoy!

PER SERVING: 64 CALORIES, 1.96G FAT, 2.57G CARBS, 6.21G PROTEIN, 0.21G FIBER, 28MG CALCIUM, 1.02MG IRON, 364MG SODIUM, 2µG FOLATE

cucumber and mint tea sandwiches

Sometimes the simplest pleasures are the best, and this little sandwich proves the point. As easy to make as it is to love, it combines the clean, refreshing flavors of cucumber and mint against the salted butter and the whole-wheat bread. Since mint can help settle a fussy stomach, these bites are also great for morning sickness. Enjoy with a warm cup of rooibos, or other caffeine-free, tea with a dash of milk.

Serves 4

2 tablespoons salted butter, softened
¼ cup finely chopped fresh mint, plus leaves for garnish
coarsely ground black pepper to taste
2 slices whole-wheat bread, crusts trimmed if desired
¼ English cucumber, peeled and sliced into thin rounds

Mix together the butter, mint, and pepper. Spread 1 tablespoon of the mint butter onto each slice of bread and top with layers of cucumber.

Slice the open-face sandwiches in half, top with a few whole mint leaves, and serve.

PER SERVING: 90 CALORIES, 5.79G FAT, 7.33G CARBS, 1.77G PROTEIN, 0.96G FIBER, 34MG CALCIUM, 1.18MG IRON, 107MG SODIUM, 18µG FOLATE

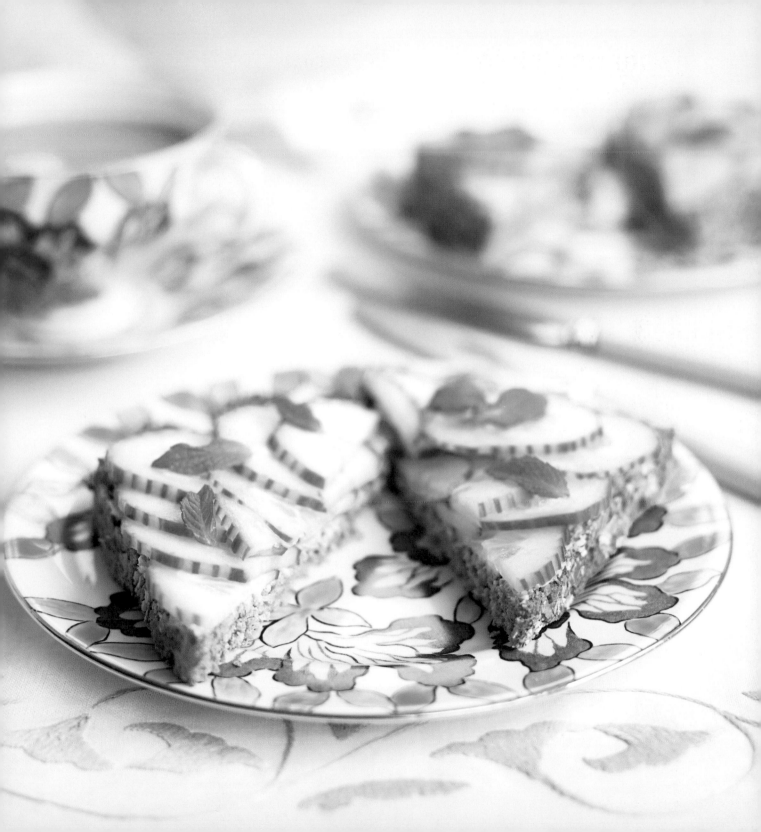

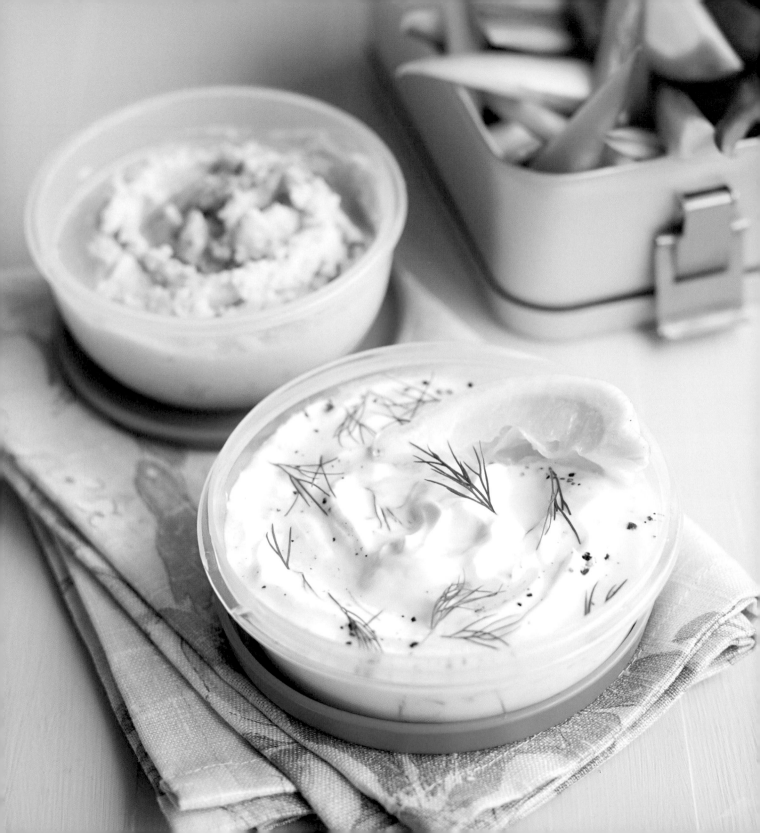

hummus and crudités

One surefire way to avoid reaching for food that's bad for you the minute you feel hungry is to keep this snack on hand at all times. Easily stored in the refrigerator, hummus with healthy things to dip in it can be a life-saver for the famished mom-to-be—and a good source of dietary fiber, protein, and folate.

Serves 8

1 tablespoon garlic, minced and mashed to a paste
½ teaspoon kosher salt
one 16-ounce can chickpeas (garbanzo beans), rinsed and drained
½ cup well-stirred tahini (sesame seed paste)
3 tablespoons fresh lemon juice
½ teaspoon white vinegar
2 tablespoons olive oil
¼ teaspoon ground cumin
2 tablespoons water
4 carrots, peeled and cut into sticks
1 cucumber, peeled and cut into sticks
2 bell peppers, cut into sticks

In a food processor, combine the garlic, salt, chickpeas, tahini, lemon juice, vinegar, oil, cumin, and water and blend until smooth. Transfer to a small serving dish.

Serve the hummus with the carrots, cucumber, and red bell peppers, or refrigerate, covered, for up to 5 days.

PER SERVING: 176 CALORIES, 7.73G FAT, 22.05G CARBS, 5.21G PROTEIN, 4.92G FIBER, 51MG CALCIUM, 1.54MG IRON, 354MG SODIUM, 73µG FOLATE

crudités with lemon-dill dip

Most creamy dips use calorie-heavy mayonnaise or sour cream as a base. But this one leverages the tangy deliciousness of Greek yogurt, making it guilt-free as well as nutritious. While you could easily devour all four servings in one sitting without concern, you can also store them in an airtight container in the refrigerator for up to three days.

Serves 4

1 cup nonfat Greek yogurt
2 tablespoons fresh dill leaves, minced
1 teaspoon fresh lemon juice
¼ teaspoon kosher salt
freshly ground black pepper to taste
4 celery stalks, sliced into sticks
1 cucumber, peeled and sliced into sticks
2 large carrots, peeled and sliced into sticks

In a small mixing bowl, mix the yogurt, dill, lemon juice, salt, and pepper until combined. Transfer to a small serving bowl and serve with the celery, cucumber, and carrots.

PER SERVING: 63 CALORIES, 0.24G FAT, 10.98G CARBS, 4.55G PROTEIN, 2.15G FIBER, 159MG CALCIUM, 0.42MG IRON, 250MG SODIUM, 38µG FOLATE

fava bean, tomato, avocado, and corn salsa

This dish is easy to prepare and perfect as a snack with toasted pita chips. It's also flexible enough that you can substitute whatever vegetables you like best (think zucchini, bell peppers, and even lightly steamed broccoli or green beans). Best of all, it's really healthy.

Serves 4

1½ pounds fava beans, unshucked
1 cup cherry tomatoes
½ firm, ripe avocado, diced
1 ear of corn (cooked or raw)
2 tablespoons extra-virgin olive oil
2 teaspoons sherry vinegar
1 tablespoon diced shallot or red onion
1 teaspoon sugar
½ teaspoon kosher salt
freshly ground black pepper

Cook the fava beans for 4 minutes in a large pot of boiling water. Drain, cool in an ice bath, and pierce and peel away the fava beans' skin. Place in a serving bowl.

Halve the tomatoes and add them to the bowl. Gently add the avocado. Cut the corn off of the cob and add.

Whisk together the olive oil, vinegar, shallot, sugar, salt, and pepper to taste.

Gently toss the salad with the dressing, add additional seasoning if necessary, and get ready for lots of praise on your culinary prowess.

PER SERVING: 280 CALORIES, 11.28G FAT, 39.35G CARBS, 15.09G PROTEIN, 2.74G FIBER, 70MG CALCIUM, 3.07MG IRON, 340MG SODIUM, 288µG FOLATE

fruit salad with orange-ginger syrup

Nausea-soothing ginger adds extra oomph to this classic, simple snack. Don't hesitate to substitute your favorite fruit or serve this over plain yogurt. Everything tastes better when coated in sweet ginger syrup!

Serves 4

⅛ cup freshly squeezed orange juice
1 tablespoon peeled and minced fresh ginger
2 tablespoons honey
½ medium cantalope, cut into bite-size chunks
1 pint ripe organic strawberries, sliced
1 cup blueberries
1 crisp red apple, cored and cut into bite-size pieces
1 cup grapes
4 mint leaves, sliced into extra-thin strips

In a small saucepan over medium heat, warm the orange juice with the ginger just until it begins to simmer, about 4 minutes.

Strain and discard the ginger, reserving the juice in a serving bowl. Mix in the honey until well combined. Add the fruit and mint, toss to evenly coat, and chill for at least 30 minutes or up to 4 hours.

PER SERVING: 162 CALORIES, 0.52G FAT, 41.50G CARBS, 2.10G PROTEIN, 5.03G FIBER, 34MG CALCIUM, 1.19MG IRON, 13MG SODIUM, 43µG FOLATE

artichokes with tarragon dip

Artichokes are a fabulous source of fiber and vitamin C, and Greek yogurt adds a shot of protein to the lemony, tarragon-tinged accompaniment. Serve these warm or cold—they're great either way.

Serves 4

1 lemon, halved
4 tablespoons low-fat mayonnaise
4 teaspoons minced fresh tarragon
2 teaspoons Dijon mustard
generous pinch freshly ground black pepper
4 tablespoons nonfat plain yogurt
4 fresh artichokes

Juice one-half of the lemon, reserving the squeezed lemon half.

In a small mixing bowl, combine the mayonnaise, tarragon, mustard, black pepper, yogurt, and 2 teaspoons lemon juice. Transfer to a small serving bowl and refrigerate, covered, for at least 30 minutes.

Fill a large pot with salted water and bring to a boil. Trim the top and bottom of each artichoke. Place the artichokes and the squeezed lemon in the boiling water, cover, and cook at a high simmer until a sharp knife goes through the bases with ease, about 30 to 45 minutes.

Drain and serve with the tarragon dip.

PER SERVING: 125 CALORIES, 5.03G FAT, 19.22G CARBS, 5.77G PROTEIN, 8.33G FIBER, 112MG CALCIUM, 2.14MG IRON, 262MG SODIUM, 90µG FOLATE

niçoise salad wheels

Fast to prepare, high in protein, niacin, and vitamin B12, and easy to store for surprise hunger attacks, this tuna-cucumber temptation is a safe snack. Just be sure to limit your intake of light tuna and other low-mercury fish to 12 ounces per week. If you prefer the taste of higher-mercury albacore tuna, drop that amount to six ounces per week. You can also swap the cucumber wheels for crackers.

Serves 4

4 teaspoons extra-virgin olive oil
2 teaspoons red wine vinegar
freshly ground black pepper
8 kalamata olives, pitted and minced
2 tablespoons minced red onion
1 (6-ounce) can light tuna packed in water
1 cucumber, peeled and sliced into sixteen
   ½-inch-thick wheels

In a nonreactive mixing bowl, combine the olive oil, vinegar, pepper, olives, and onion. Set aside for 15 minutes.

Drain the canned tuna, transfer to a small serving bowl, and add the vinaigrette. Gently stir to combine.

Serve with the cucumber wheels.

PER SERVING: 73 CALORIES, 5.29G FAT, 2.01G CARBS, 4.13G PROTEIN, 0.73G FIBER, 14MG CALCIUM, 0.46MG IRON, 133MG SODIUM, 10µG FOLATE

margherita toast

Have your pizza and eat it too with this single-serving taste of Italy. Easy to prepare and a better bet than a whole pie for those seeking help with portion control, it can also be customized to your liking—just add sliced mushrooms, olives, chopped bell pepper, pineapple, or anything else you like.

Serves 1

1 tablespoon marinara sauce
½ whole-grain English muffin or slice of bread, toasted
1 thin slice low-fat mozzarella
5 basil leaves

Preheat the broiler (alternately, use a toaster oven).

Spread the marinara sauce on the English muffin half. Top with the cheese and basil. Broil, or toast, until the cheese is melted, about 5 minutes.

PER SERVING: 163 CALORIES, 6.29G FAT, 16.68G CARBS, 10.54G PROTEIN, 2.67G FIBER, 298MG CALCIUM, 1.07MG IRON, 367MG SODIUM, 21µG FOLATE

not-so-naughty nachos

The key to success with this health-friendly version of classic nachos is to make sure you've got friends to help you polish off the plate. Or just make one-quarter of the recipe when snacking solo so you don't overeat.

Serves 4

18 baked tortilla chips (about 1 ounce)
½ cup loosely packed shredded Cheddar
  and Monterey Jack cheese
1 heaping tablespoon seeded and diced ripe red tomato
⅛ cup small diced firm avocado
1 tablespoon sliced green onion
1 tablespoon canned "nacho sliced" jalapeños, chopped
kosher salt

Preheat the broiler.

Scatter the chips on a baking sheet covered with foil. Sprinkle the cheese on top of the chips and broil in the middle of the oven, until the cheese is just melted, about 3 to 4 minutes.

Sprinkle the tomato, avocado, green onion, jalapeño, and a dash of salt over the nachos and serve.

PER SERVING: 102 CALORIES, 5.74G FAT, 7.80G CARBS, 4.74G PROTEIN, 1.26G FIBER, 118MG CALCIUM, 0.39MG IRON, 154MG SODIUM, 14µG FOLATE

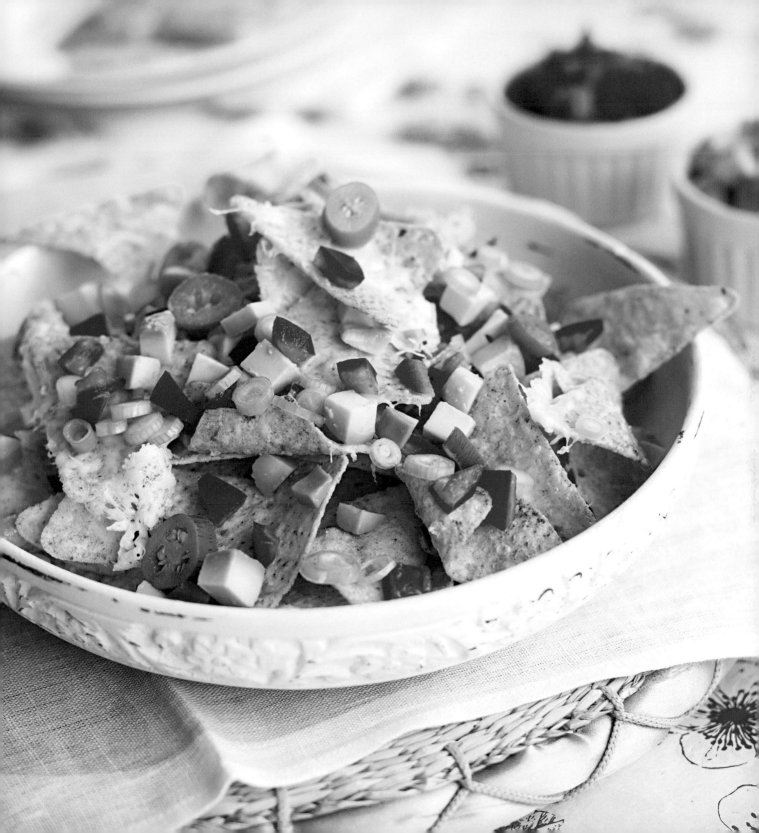

grilled cheese sandwich gone good

While nothing beats the classic butter-saturated sandwich fully loaded with melted American, fontina, or Gruyère, there is a healthier way to get your grease on. And this sandwich is it. Want to gussy it up? Go ahead and add a slice of tomato, ham, or both before cooking. You deserve it!

Serves 1

½ teaspoon extra-virgin olive oil
2 slices of whole-wheat bread
1 thick slice of Cheddar, mozzarella, or Monterey Jack

Preheat the oven to 350°F.

Heat the olive oil in a small oven-safe skillet over medium heat, tilting the pan so the oil evenly coats the bottom, until hot but not smoking. Add a slice of bread, layer with the cheese and the second slice of bread. Cook the sandwich until the bottom is crisp and golden, about 2 minutes, then flip to toast the other side.

Transfer to the oven for 5 to 7 minutes, or until the cheese is melted. Enjoy!

PER SERVING: 264 CALORIES, 12.52G FAT, 24.11G CARBS, 12.43G PROTEIN, 1.80G FIBER, 272MG CALCIUM, 1.93MG IRON, 433MG SODIUM, 47µG FOLATE

herbed parmesan popcorn

While popcorn isn't exactly the pinnacle of nutrition, it is a fantastically light snack when prepared without gobs of oil or butter. Incidentally, you can change up these toppings quite easily – just swap the cheese and parsley for curry powder, nutritional yeast, or garlic powder.

Serves 1

olive oil spray
3 cups of air-popped popcorn
2 tablespoons freshly grated Parmesan cheese
¼ teaspoon kosher salt
½ teaspoon dried parsley

Lightly spray the popcorn with olive oil, add the cheese, salt, and parsley, and toss until combined. Serve.

PER SERVING: 118 CALORIES, 2.61G FAT, 19.05G CARBS, 5.48G PROTEIN, 3.70G FIBER, 89MG CALCIUM, 0.95MG IRON, 696MG SODIUM, 5µG FOLATE

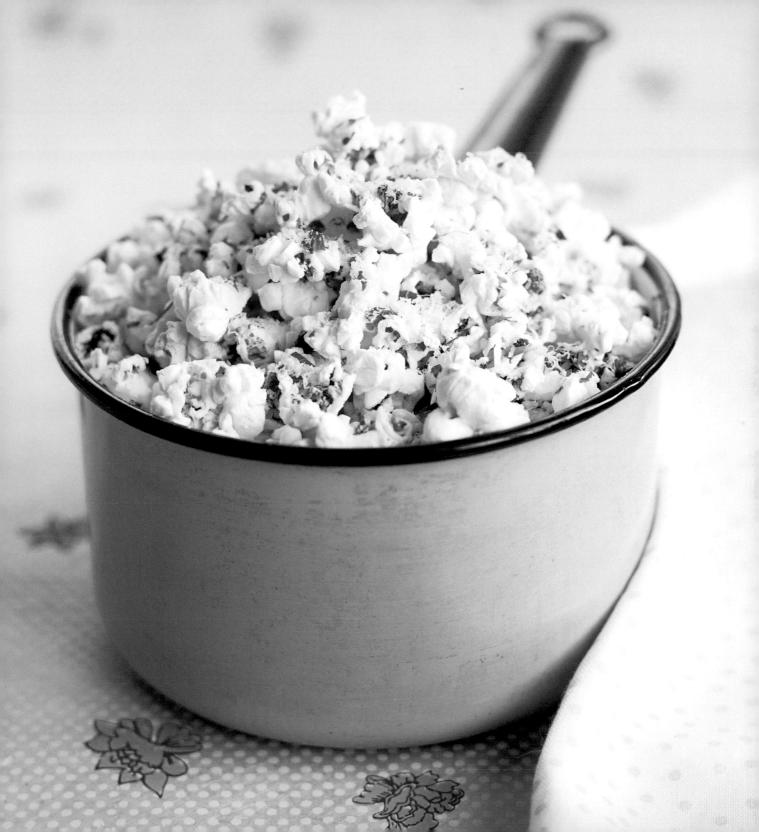

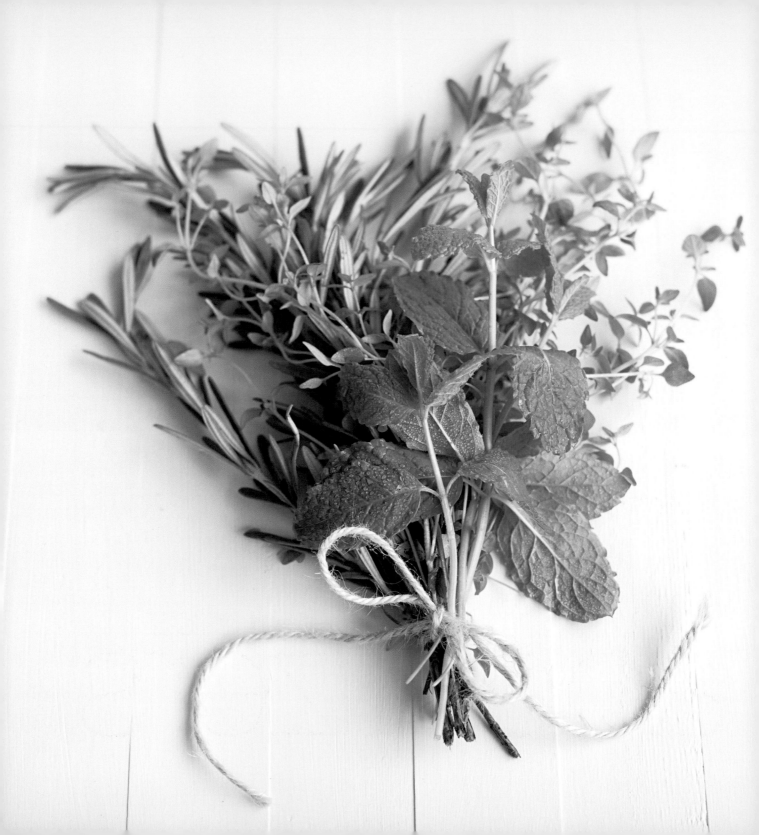

chapter three
appetizers

craigie on main maine mussels

This contribution from Tony Maws, two-time James Beard Award-nominated chef and owner of the heralded restaurant Craigie on Main, is pure genius. Not only is it ridiculously easy and quick to prepare, but its broth is a startlingly exceptional and exotic diversion from white wine–based preparations. The dish is also a fine source of protein, iron, copper, and selenium. Add some grilled crusty bread for dipping and you've found nirvana.

Serves 4

2 tablespoons extra-virgin olive oil
1 clove garlic, slivered
12 mussels (about ½ pound), cleaned and
    beards removed
pinch of coarse gray sea, or kosher, salt
pinch of New Mexican red chile caribe or
    red chile flakes
small pinch of high-quality saffron
1 teaspoon pastis
1 tablespoon sake
1½ teaspoons yellow miso
1½ teaspoon unsalted butter, softened
1 tablespoon vegetable stock
1 tablespoon chopped herbs (parsley,
    tarragon, chervil, tarragon)
¾ teaspoon fresh lemon juice

Gently heat 1 tablespoon olive oil and the garlic in a heavy-bottomed pan over medium-high heat until the garlic toasts, becoming golden but not any darker. Remove the garlic from the pan with a slotted spoon and set aside.

Place the mussels in the infused olive oil and add the sea salt, chile, and saffron. Roast the mussels in the pan until they begin to open, then transfer them with the slotted spoon to a large bowl. Discard any mussels that don't open.

Deglaze the pan with the pastis and sake. Mix the miso and butter together and add it to the pan along with the vegetable stock and the reserved cooked garlic. Cook until the butter melts. Finish with the chopped herbs, lemon juice, and remaining 1 tablespoon olive oil. Divide the sauce and mussels among four shallow bowls and serve.

PER SERVING: 124 CALORIES, 8.77G FAT, 3.16G CARBS, 6.10G PROTEIN, 0.25G FIBER, 16MG CALCIUM, 2.09MG IRON, 304MG SODIUM, 23µG FOLATE

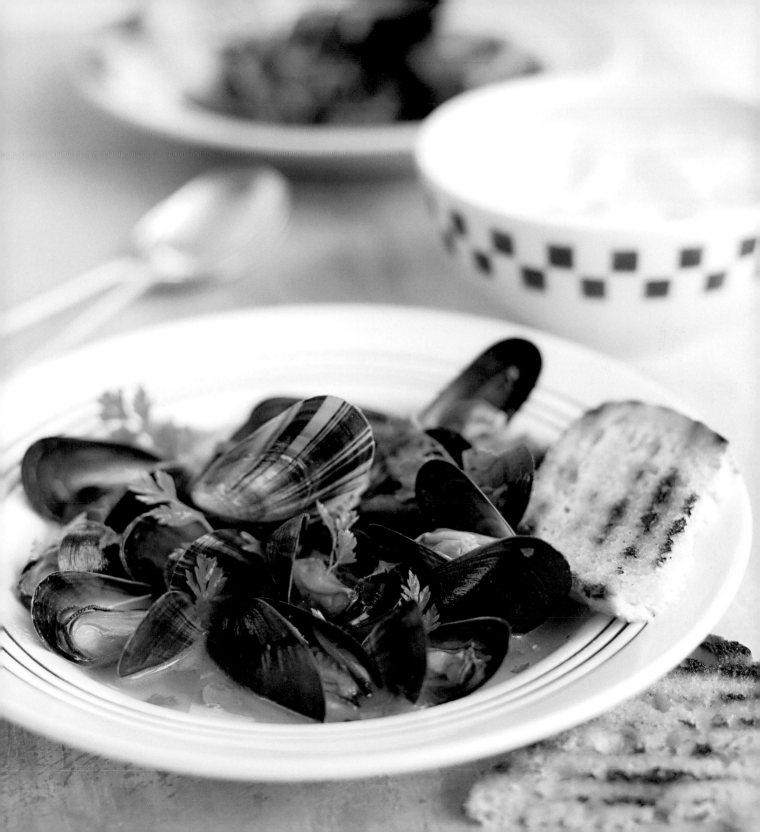

deviled egg-salad bites

These irresistible two-bite crowd-pleasers are classics with a crunchy celery twist. They are also fast and easy sources of protein.

Serves 4

2 hard-boiled eggs, halved
1 tablespoon mayonnaise
1/8 teaspoon hot dry mustard powder
1/8 teaspoon kosher salt
1 tablespoon minced celery
paprika
1/2 teaspoon minced chives (optional)

Carefully remove the yolks from the eggs, transfer to a small mixing bowl, and mash with the back of a fork until broken into small bits. Stir in the mayonnaise, mustard powder, and salt until well combined. Fold in the celery.

Scoop the mixture into the egg whites, sprinkle with paprika and chives, if desired, and serve.

PER SERVING: 62 CALORIES, 4.89G FAT, 0.30G CARBS, 3.19G PROTEIN, 0.05G FIBER, 14MG CALCIUM, 0.48MG IRON, 127MG SODIUM, 12μG FOLATE

baked pot stickers

These tiny purses of seasoned pork and shrimp are as good as those served in Chinese restaurants, but because they are baked instead of fried, they are far less greasy. If you don't have mini cupcake pans, fold the wonton wrappers tortellini-style and bake them on a baking sheet.

Makes 24

1/2 pound ground pork
10 medium shrimp, peeled, deveined, and chopped
1 teaspoon minced garlic
1 tablespoon finely chopped fresh ginger
3 tablespoons finely chopped green onions
1/4 cup finely chopped canned water chestnuts
1 egg yolk
2 teaspoons low-sodium soy sauce, plus more for serving
1 1/2 teaspoons rice wine vinegar
1/2 teaspoon unseasoned sesame oil
24 wonton wrappers
Chinese hot sauce (optional), for serving

Preheat the oven to 400°F.

In a small mixing bowl combine all of the ingredients except the wrappers and hot sauce and mix until thoroughly combined. Working on a flat work surface, lay out a few of the wonton wrappers. (Keep the rest covered with plastic wrap.) Place a heaping teaspoon of the filling in the center of each wonton wrapper. Lightly wet your fingers with water, then wet the edges of the wonton, pressing the edges together. Transfer, edges facing up, to a mini cupcake pan. Repeat until two cupcake pans are full. (Or make in two batches.)

Bake for 10 minutes or until the wonton juices are bubbling. Serve with soy sauce and hot sauce.

PER POT STICKER: 55 CALORIES, 2.21G FAT, 5.03G CARBS, 3.09G PROTEIN, 0.21G FIBER, 8MG CALCIUM, 0.47MG IRON, 69MG SODIUM, 9μG FOLATE

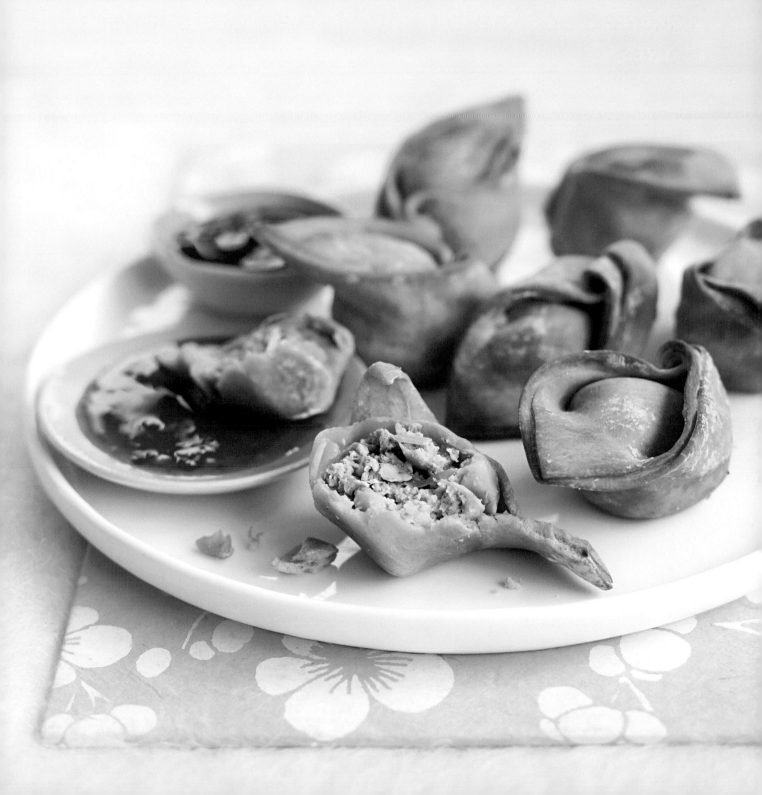

classic california hand rolls

While the potential of contracting listeria from raw fish causes many OB-GYNs to warn pregnant women against indulging in most options, not all sushi is off the table. You can easily and safely satisfy cravings by whipping up these hand rolls. You can also substitute other fillings, such as cooked asparagus, green beans, shrimp, scallops, or mango spears. Regardless, serve them with the expected accompaniments of soy sauce and wasabi (available in powder form in many markets).

Makes 6 hand rolls

¾ cups sushi rice
1 cup water
⅓ pound (about ¾ cup) fresh or frozen crabmeat
1 tablespoon mayonnaise
2 tablespoons unseasoned rice wine vinegar
2 teaspoons sugar
¾ teaspoon kosher salt
3 sheets of nori (available at Asian specialty markets)
¼ teaspoon toasted sesame seeds
6 (3 x ½-inch) cucumber spears
½ ripe Hass avocado, sliced thinly

Rinse the rice multiple times, until the water is clear. Drain and transfer to a saucepan with a tight-sealing lid. Add the water, place on high heat, and bring to a boil. Cover the pot, reduce the flame, and simmer for 20 minutes.

Meanwhile, in another small bowl, combine the vinegar, sugar, and salt. Transfer the cooked rice to a large mixing bowl and add the vinegar mixture. Using a rubber spatula, gently mix. Cool the rice to just warm and cover with a clean damp dish towel.

In a small bowl, mix the crab and mayonnaise; set aside.

Cut the 3 nori sheets in half crosswise. Set one half down, with the short sides facing you, on a flat surface. Using moistened hands, gently press down a little less than ¼ cup of cooked rice onto the bottom half of the nori sheet. Sprinkle the rice with sesame seeds, top with a cucumber spear, add 1 thin slice of avocado, and 1 tablespoon crab mixture. Holding the rice-covered part of the nori in the palm of your hand, fold the uncovered half of the nori over the fillings into a cone shape.

Repeat with the remaining ingredients until you have 6 hand rolls. Serve.

PER SERVING: 100 CALORIES, 4.50G FAT, 8.98G CARBS, 5.59G PROTEIN, 1.39G FIBER, 31MG CALCIUM, 0.61MG IRON, 19MG SODIUM, 39µG FOLATE

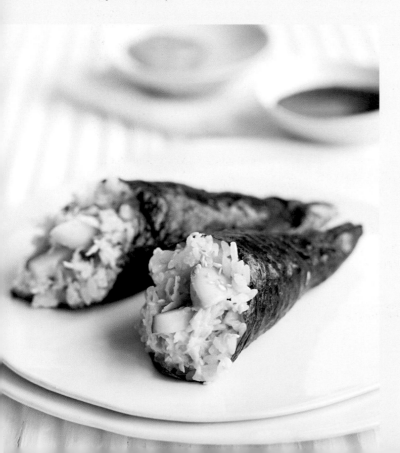

balinese chicken satays with peanut sauce

Unlike ubiquitous "satays," which consist of thinly sliced chicken on a skewer, this exotic Balinese-style appetizer, based on a recipe from the Four Season resort at Sayan in Bali, is a mixture of ground chicken and Southeast Asian spices served on a lemongrass stick. Note: If you can't find kaffir lime leaves, add half of a bay leaf when cooking the spices, then remove it and add a generous pinch of lime zest when you add the coconut.

Serves 4

3 teaspoons canola oil
1 tablespoon plus 1 teaspoon
  minced garlic
¼ teaspoon red pepper flakes
3½ teaspoons minced fresh ginger
½ teaspoon turmeric
⅛ teaspoon ground white pepper
1 clove, crushed
½ teaspoon ground nutmeg
½ teaspoon ground coriander
½ teaspoon kosher salt
1 pound ground chicken
1 kaffir lime leaf, finely shredded
¼ cup grated, unsweetened coconut
kosher salt and freshly ground
  black pepper
4 lemongrass stalks, halved
2 tablespoons plus 1 teaspoon
  minced shallots
2 teaspoons brown sugar
2 teaspoons fresh lime juice
½ cup creamy peanut butter
4 tablespoons water

Preheat the oven to 400°F. Line a baking sheet with parchment paper.

In a small sauté pan, heat 2 teaspoons oil over low heat. Add 1 tablespoon garlic, ⅛ teaspoon red pepper flakes, 2 teaspoons ginger, the turmeric, white pepper, clove, nutmeg, coriander, and salt and sauté until aromatic and cooked, about 5 minutes. Remove from the heat, cool, and transfer to a medium mixing bowl. Mash to a paste with the back of a spoon, then mix in the ground chicken, lime leaf, and coconut until completely combined. Season with salt and pepper.

Take ⅛ of the chicken mixture and mold it around the top half of a lemongrass "skewer" so that it's shaped like a narrow popsicle. Transfer to the lined baking sheet. Repeat with all the lemongrass and chicken, making sure they are evenly spaced on the baking sheet. Bake for 15 to 20 minutes or until cooked through.

Meanwhile, make the peanut sauce. In a small sauté pan over medium heat, heat 1 teaspoon oil until hot but not smoking. Add the shallot, 1 teaspoon garlic, ⅛ teaspoon red pepper flakes, and 1½ teaspoons ginger and cook until aromatic.

Add the brown sugar, lime juice, peanut butter, and water and stir to combine, adding more water if the consistency is too thick. Transfer to a serving bowl and serve at room temperature or store, refrigerated and covered, up to 3 days.

PER SERVING: 213 CALORIES, 14.91G FAT, 6.48G CARBS, 14.34G PROTEIN, 1.47G FIBER, 18MG CALCIUM, 1.21MG IRON, 255MG SODIUM, 15µG FOLATE

minced chicken lettuce wraps

This classic and beloved Chinese appetizer is high in protein, low in carbs (which is great for anyone struggling with gestational diabetes), and a good source of potassium and vitamin D, thanks to the mushrooms. It's also as fun to eat as it is flavorful. Just serve the minced chicken in a decorative bowl with a side of stacked lettuce leaves and let diners build their own Asian-style burritos. Or make a batch for yourself and save the extra helpings for future snacking.

Serves 4

1 pound boneless skinless chicken breast
2 teaspoons vegetable oil
1 (5-ounce) can water chestnuts, drained and minced
2/3 cup diced fresh shiitake or cremini mushrooms
1 carrot, minced (about ½ cup)
1 stalk celery, minced (about ¼ cup)
1 tablespoon minced fresh garlic
2 tablespoons low-sodium soy sauce
2 tablespoons brown sugar
4 teaspoons seasoned rice vinegar
2 tablespoons sliced green onions
8 large iceberg lettuce leaves

Preheat the oven to 350°F. Rub the chicken breast with 1 teaspoon oil and bake in an oven-safe sauté pan for 30 minutes or until cooked through. Carefully transfer the chicken to a plate to cool.

Add another teaspoon of oil to the sauté pan and heat on the stove top over medium heat until hot but not smoking, then add the water chestnuts, mushrooms, carrot, celery, and garlic. Sauté, stirring frequently, for 3 minutes. Finely chop the cooled chicken and add it to the vegetables.

In a small bowl, mix the soy sauce, sugar, and vinegar, add it to the chicken and vegetables, and sauté over medium-high heat, stirring frequently, for 2 minutes. Transfer the mixture to a serving bowl and serve with a side stack of lettuce "cups."

To eat, place a scoop of minced chicken in the center of a lettuce leaf, wrap the lettuce around its filling, and enjoy!

PER SERVING: 207 CALORIES, 3.38G FAT, 14.31G CARBS, 28.14G PROTEIN, 2.60G FIBER, 38MG CALCIUM, 1.68MG IRON, 367MG SODIUM, 26μG FOLATE

shrimp, avocado, and mango cocktail with cilantro-lime dressing

If any recipe proves that elegance is all in the presentation, this one is it. Ridiculously quick to prepare, bright and fresh in flavor and color, and imparting potassium and vitamins C and B6, it becomes downright glamorous when served in a juice or cocktail glass.

Serves 4

2 teaspoons fresh lime juice
4 teaspoons extra-virgin olive oil
3 tablespoons chopped fresh cilantro, plus 4 sprigs for garnish
¼ teaspoon honey
⅛ teaspoon kosher salt
4 romaine lettuce leaves, sliced crosswise into ¾-inch strips
½ Hass avocado, cubed
½ mango, cubed
12 shrimp, peeled, deveined, cooked, and chopped, plus 4 kept whole

In a blender, combine the lime juice, olive oil, cilantro, honey, and salt, and blend for 30 seconds or until the cilantro is liquefied. Set aside.

Using 4 juice or martini glasses, place ¼ of the shredded lettuce at the bottom of each glass. Add a layer of avocado, mango, chopped shrimp, and a drizzle of dressing. Finish by adding a sprig of cilantro and one whole cooked shrimp to each glass.

PER SERVING: 122 CALORIES, 8.17G FAT, 8.21G CARBS, 4.65G PROTEIN, 2.76G FIBER, 24MG CALCIUM, 0.91MG IRON, 30MG SODIUM, 62µG FOLATE

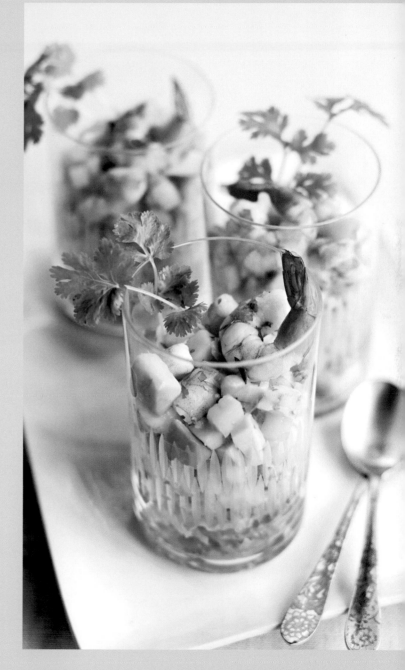

eggplant caprese napoleons

So simple, so fresh, and so good for you, this beautiful first course could easily act as a light lunch, too. Just grill extra eggplant and store it in the fridge so you can effortlessly make it anytime. Also, you can easily broil the eggplant instead of grilling it; place it on a broiler pan—not too close to the flame—baste with oil and toast both sides, watching carefully so it doesn't burn.

Serves 4

1 large eggplant
¼ teaspoon kosher salt, plus a little more to finish
1 clove garlic, pressed or minced
2 tablespoons olive oil
1 large heirloom or other flavorful, ripe tomato, cut into 4 slices
4 ounces pasteurized buffalo mozzarella cheese, cut into 4 slices
¼ cup balsamic vinegar
¼ cup fresh basil leaves
freshly cracked black pepper

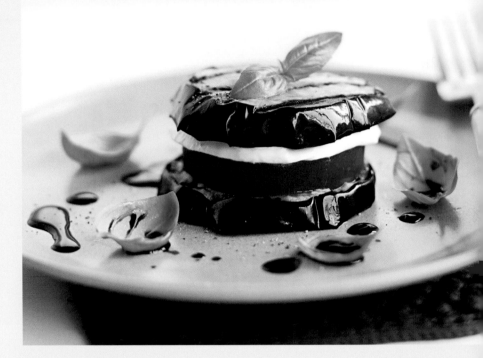

Preheat the grill. Slice off and discard the top and bottom of the eggplant and slice the remainder into 8 slices. Season with the salt and let sit for 10 minutes.

Mix the olive oil and garlic in a small bowl. Using a basting brush or spoon, brush the eggplant with the garlic oil. Grill the eggplant until golden on both sides, about 8 minutes total.

On a serving platter, arrange 4 grilled eggplant discs. Top with a layer of tomato, a layer of mozzarella, and a final layer of eggplant. Set aside.

In a small saucepan over medium-high heat, bring the vinegar to a boil and reduce to a syrup, watching carefully not to burn it, about 4 minutes. Carefully drizzle the syrup over the 4 napoleons, adding extra drops on the platter for decoration. Sprinkle the basil atop the stacks and around the platter and sprinkle with salt and cracked pepper. Serve.

PER SERVING: 206 CALORIES, 13.44G FAT, 13.29G CARBS, 8.08G PROTEIN, 5.24G FIBER, 187MG CALCIUM, 0.72MG IRON, 271MG SODIUM, 40µG FOLATE

stewed tomato and white bean bruschetta

The secret to the full, rustic deliciousness of this Italian-style appetizer is in the sauce, so be sure to use vine-ripened tomatoes (ideally in summertime) for optimal flavor. Also, there's no need to wait for dining companions to make this recipe. Single servings come easily if you prepare and refrigerate the beans with sauce and return to it whenever you want to adorn a piece of toast.

Serves 4

1 tablespoon extra-virgin olive oil
2 cloves garlic
2 large vine-ripened tomatoes, peeled, cut into 6 pieces and seeded
generous pinch red pepper flakes
½ teaspoon kosher salt
generous pinch freshly ground black pepper
⅓ cup chopped basil
¾ cup cooked white beans, drained and rinsed
4 thin slices crusty Italian bread or 8 thin baguette slices
¼ cup pasteurized feta, crumbled

In a wide pan, heat the olive oil over medium-high heat. Crush 1 clove of garlic and add to the pan. Add the garlic, tomatoes, red pepper flakes, salt, and black pepper. Cook for 5 minutes or until the tomatoes start to soften.

Using a potato masher, smash the tomatoes. Continue cooking until the tomatoes become a thick sauce and there is very little liquid remaining, about 10 to 15 minutes. Stir in the basil and white beans.

Meanwhile, preheat the broiler. (Alternately, use a toaster oven.) Rub one side of each slice of bread with the remaining garlic clove. Transfer to a broiler-safe pan, garlic-side up, and toast the bread until golden. Top with the bean and tomato mixture and crumbled feta and broil until hot, about 5 minutes, watching to make sure it doesn't burn.

Serve warm or at room temperature.

PER SERVING: 139 CALORIES, 5.74G FAT, 16.54G CARBS, 5.94G PROTEIN, 3.77G FIBER, 91MG CALCIUM, 1.44MG IRON, 458MG SODIUM, 70µG FOLATE

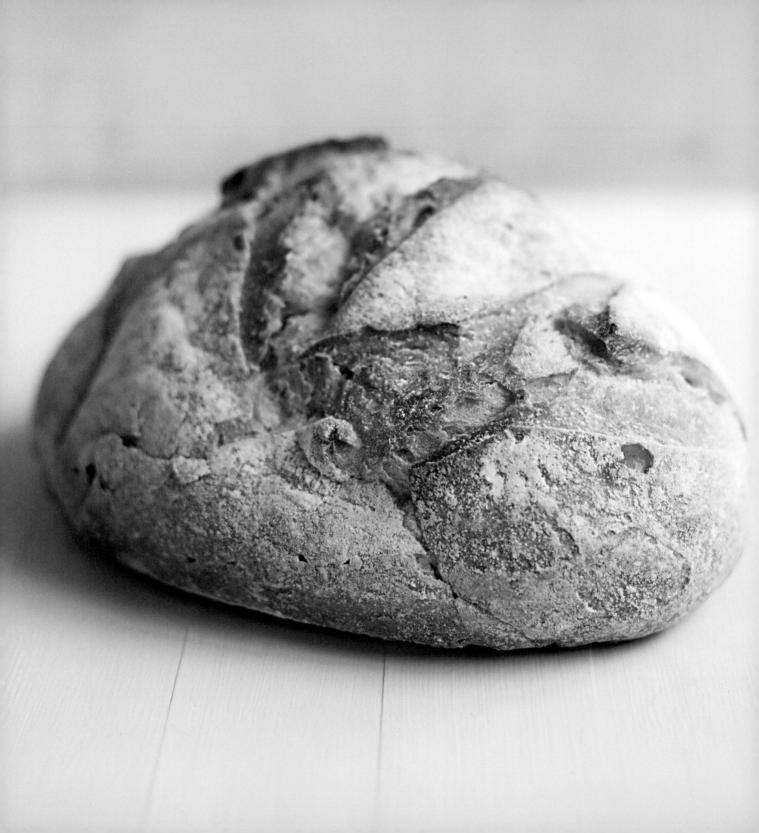

chapter four

soups & salads

gazpacho with shrimp

When invited to ante up a pregnancy-friendly dish for this book, Washington, D.C.'s famed chef José Andrés forwarded this recipe, an adaptation of his wife Patricia Fernandez de la Cruz's gazpacho. Loaded with fresh vegetables and topped with shrimp, it's a light yet filling meal. And because it's served chilled, it's also soothing to the overheated mom-to-be.

Serves 4

For the gazpacho
2 pounds ripe tomatoes, peeled, seeded, and diced
½ cucumber, peeled, seeded, and diced
½ green pepper, seeded and diced
1 cup water
6 tablespoons extra-virgin olive oil
2 tablespoons sherry vinegar
1 to 1½ slices of bread, torn into small pieces
½ teaspoon kosher salt

For the shrimp
12 large shrimp, peeled and deveined
1 tablespoon olive oil
pinch of kosher salt

For the garnish
4 (½-inch thick) slices of bread, cut into ½-inch cubes
1 tablespoon olive oil
4 plum tomatoes, peeled, seeded and diced
½ cucumber, peeled, seeded and diced
kosher salt, as needed
½ red bell pepper, seeded and diced
½ green bell pepper, seeded and diced
1 tablespoon diced shallot
1 tablespoon minced chives, to garnish
sea salt, to garnish

Place the gazpacho ingredients in a blender and blend until very smooth, adding more water if necessary. Strain through a fine-mesh sieve and chill.

Make the shrimp: Heat the oil in a large skillet over medium-high heat. Cut the shrimp lengthwise about halfway down so they open into a Y shape (this allows the shrimp to cook more evenly.) Once the oil is hot, sauté the shrimp for 2 to 3 minutes. Set aside.

Preheat the oven to 350°F. Put the bread cubes in a mixing bowl, drizzle with 1 tablespoon olive oil, and toss to coat evenly. Spread the cubes in a single layer on a baking sheet and bake until golden, turning once or twice with a spatula, 15 to 20 minutes. Let cool.

In a mixing bowl, combine the plum tomatoes, cucumber, red and green bell peppers, and shallot and mix well.

To serve, place three sautéed shrimp in the center of four soup bowls. Arrange some of the tomato-cucumber mixture around the edge. Sprinkle with chives and sea salt and top with some croutons. Drizzle with a little extra-virgin olive oil. Pour the chilled gazpacho into a pitcher. Set the bowls in front of your guests and pour some of the gazpacho at the table.

PER SERVING: 384 CALORIES, 28.55G FAT, 22.68G CARBS, 9.53G PROTEIN, 5.16G FIBER, 68MG CALCIUM, 2.32MG IRON, 426MG SODIUM, 90µG FOLATE

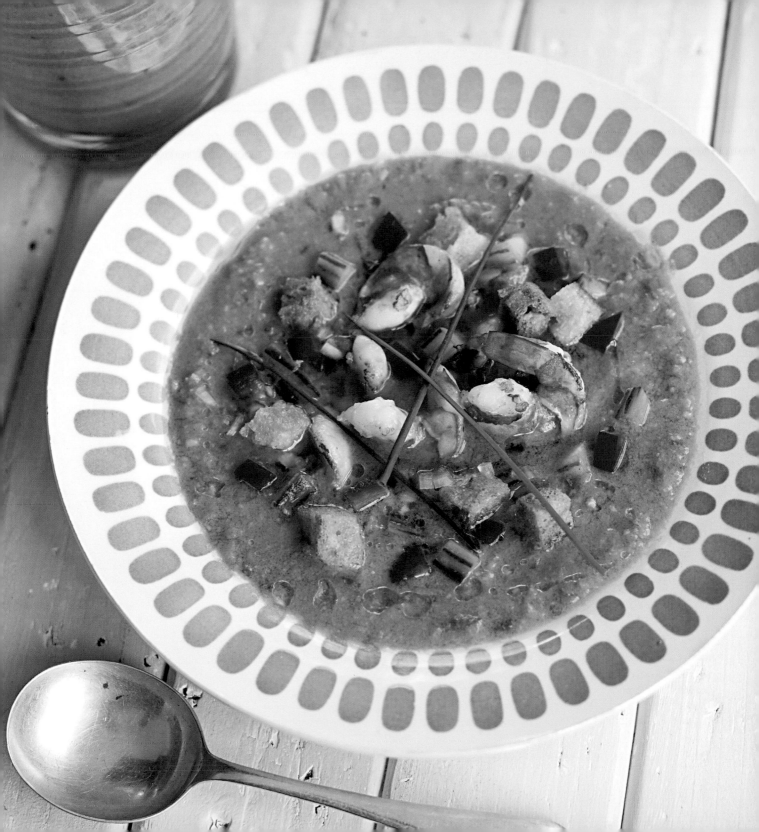

decadent chicken soup

Chicken soup is not only delicious and nutritious, but also aids in curing colds and flu—a perk for someone who's steering clear of medications for the sake of her unborn baby. The addition of onion to this dish gives it a richness reminiscent of French onion soup (minus the calories) and the veggies impart added nutritional benefit. Double the recipe and freeze it for future consumption.

Serves 4

6 cups water
½ chicken, with bones, cut into pieces
2 whole yellow onions, unpeeled
1 parsnip, peeled
1 rutabaga, peeled and quartered
1 large turnip, peeled and quartered
salt and freshly ground black pepper
½ zucchini, diced
½ carrot, diced

Put the water and chicken in a large pot and bring to a boil. Skim off any white froth that rises to the top. Add the onions, parsnip, rutabaga, and turnip, cover, and simmer for at least 2½ hours.

Remove from the heat and let cool. Remove the chicken, discard the vegetables, and strain the broth into a clean pot.

Remove and discard the skin and bones from the chicken, cut the meat into bite-size chunks, and add back to the pot. Season with salt and pepper then bring to a boil. Add the zucchini and carrot, simmer 10 minutes, or until the vegetables are cooked but are still firm, and serve hot.

PER SERVING: 135 CALORIES, 1.45G FAT, 23.46G CARBS, 8.30G PROTEIN, 6.28G FIBER, 102MG CALCIUM, 1.29MG IRON, 90MG SODIUM, 68µG FOLATE

hot and sour chicken and shrimp soup

The genius of this Thai-style soup is it is lightning-fast to prepare and amazingly light, yet boldly flavorful. It's also quite flexible. Skip the chicken, shrimp, or both, or add broccoli, bok choy, or spinach if you desire. The number of combinations is limited only by your imagination and refrigerator contents. Bonus: The soup's spices can help clear pregnancy-related congestion.

Serves 4

6 cups chicken broth
¾ pound boneless, skinless chicken, thinly sliced
    into 2 x 1-inch strips
12 shrimp, peeled and deveined
1½ cups sliced cremini or other mushrooms
2 tablespoons thinly sliced fresh lemongrass
2 tablespoons minced fresh ginger
1 to 2 fresh, hot bird's eye or other chile, minced
3 to 4 tablespoons fish sauce
3 tablespoons lime juice

In a large pot bring the chicken broth to a boil. Add the chicken, shrimp, mushrooms, lemongrass, ginger, and chile pepper and cook until the chicken is just cooked through, about 3 minutes.

Season with the fish sauce and lime juice, adding more if desired.

Ladle into 4 bowls and serve.

PER SERVING: 272 CALORIES, 5.21G FAT, 18.42G CARBS, 35.11G PROTEIN, 0.92G FIBER, 39MG CALCIUM, 2.71MG IRON, 1353MG SODIUM, 32µG FOLATE

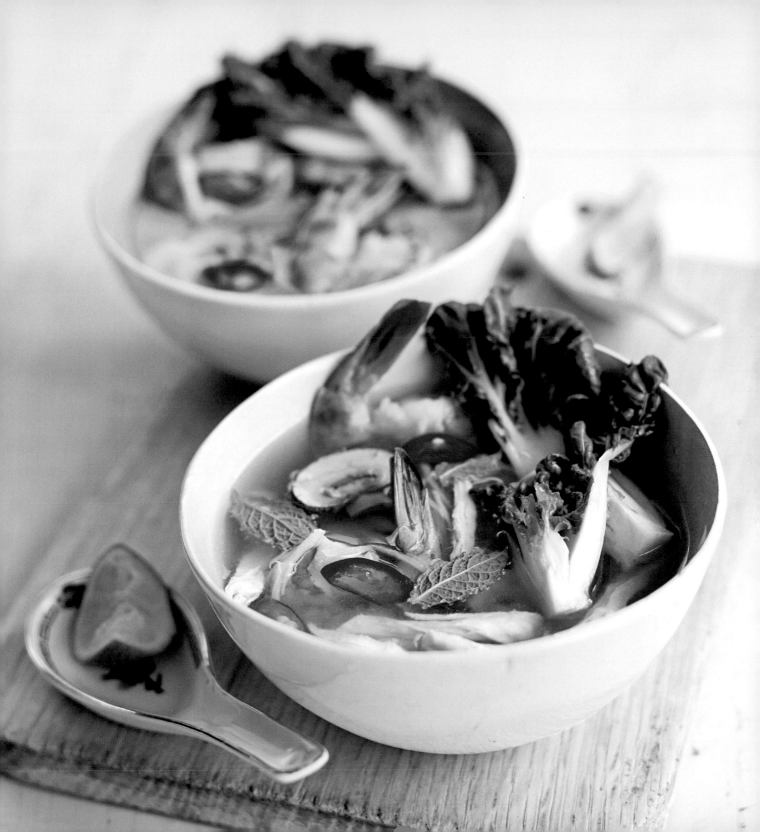

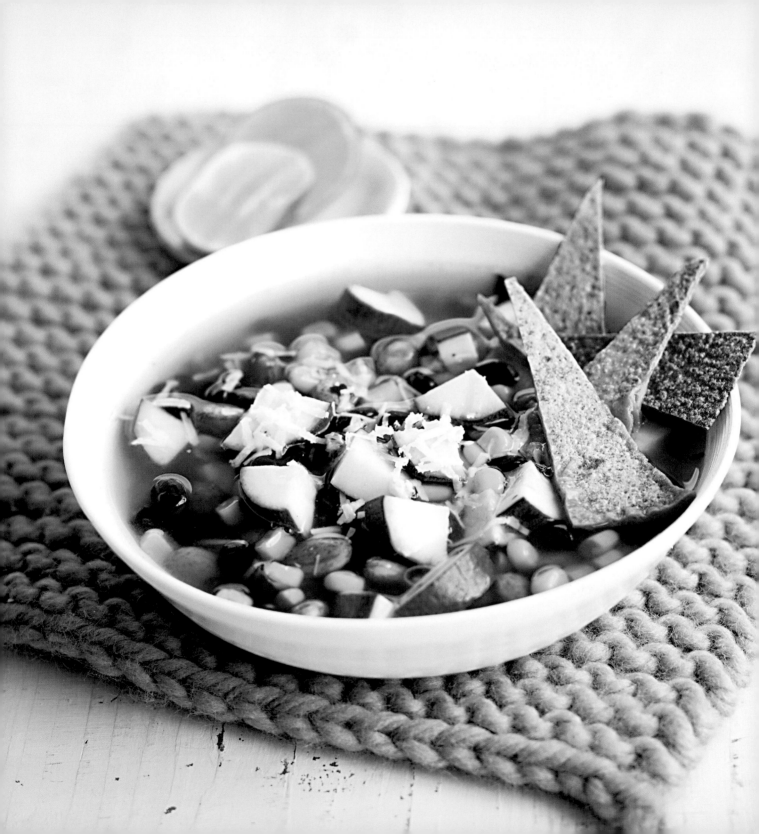

southwestern bean and vegetable soup

carrot-ginger soup

If you're craving Mexican food, don't reach for fast-food tacos. Instead, try this soup. Its spices conjure the flavor of seasoned ground beef and the beans add heartiness (not to mention much-needed fiber and protein), but its light, vegetarian nature means it's far better for you.

Easy to prepare and perfect for a light lunch, dinner, or between-meal snack, this recipe by New York food writer and chef Lisa Roberts-Lehan offers comfort in the form of stomach-settling ginger. It also boasts vitamin K–rich carrots, and leeks, onions, and garlic, which reduce "bad" cholesterol.

Serves 6

2 (6-inch) corn tortillas
6 cups chicken or vegetable broth
1 (15-ounce) pinto beans, rinsed and drained
1 (15-ounce) can black beans, rinsed and drained
1 (15-ounce) can corn, rinsed and drained
2 medium zucchini, quartered lengthwise and cut into slices
¾ teaspoon dried oregano
½ teaspoon ground cumin
¾ teaspoon paprika
¼ teaspoon chili powder
⅛ teaspoon hot red pepper flakes
½ teaspoon kosher salt
1 teaspoon lime juice plus 1 lime, cut into 6 wedges
½ cup Cheddar, grated (optional)

Serves 4

3 tablespoons olive oil
1 small onion, diced (about 2 cups)
1 leek, white part only, chopped
2 tablespoons ginger, peeled and sliced thinly (add more to taste)
2 cloves of garlic, chopped
4 cups vegetable broth
1 cup low-fat milk or unsweetened almond milk
freshly ground black pepper
1½ bunches carrots (about 9 to 12 medium carrots), stemmed, peeled, and chopped
½ teaspoon kosher salt

Preheat the oven to 350°F. Slice the tortillas into ⅓-inch-wide strips, then halve them. Spread in a single layer on a baking sheet and bake for 20 minutes or until crisp. Let cool.

In a stockpot, combine the broth, beans, corn, zucchini, and spices. Bring to a boil, then reduce to a simmer and cook for 5 minutes. Stir in the lime juice.

Ladle the soup into 6 bowls, top with tortilla strips and Cheddar. Serve with a lime wedge on the side.

In a large soup pot, heat the oil over medium heat. Add the onion, leek, ginger, and garlic and sauté for 1 to 2 minutes. Add the broth, milk, pepper, carrots, and salt. Bring to a simmer and cook until the carrots are soft, about 20 to 30 minutes, or until tender.

Remove the pot from the heat and let the soup cool for 3 to 5 minutes. Place the soup in a blender, blend until smooth, adding more water if needed. Once all the soup is blended, return to the pot and simmer to reheat.

PER SERVING: 221 CALORIES, 10.86G FAT, 27.85G CARBS, 4.34G PROTEIN, 5.34G FIBER, 145MG CALCIUM, 1.38MG IRON, 1367MG SODIUM, 50µG FOLATE

PER SERVING: 345 CALORIES, 6.97G FAT, 52.38G CARBS, 20.75G PROTEIN, 12.22G FIBER, 140MG CALCIUM, 3.83MG IRON, 887MG SODIUM, 228µG FOLATE

chopped vegetable salad with avocado and parmesan

San Francisco chef David Gingrass garnered legions of fans with this simple, yet wholly satisfying and abundantly healthful salad. Add roasted chicken for extra protein and substance.

Serves 4

1 small shallot, minced
½ teaspoon Dijon mustard
1 tablespoon sherry wine vinegar
2 tablespoons extra-virgin olive oil, plus more for salad
kosher salt and freshly ground black pepper
½ ripe avocado, diced
1 cup fresh corn kernels (or other sweet vegetable in season such as peas, fava beans, or squash)
¼ cup diced red onions
¼ cup diced blanched carrots
¼ cup diced celery hearts
½ cup seeded and diced English cucumbers
1 cup chopped mixed greens
½ cup halved cherry tomatoes
¼ cup grated Parmesan

Combine the shallot, mustard, and vinegar and mix well. Whisk in the oil. Season to taste with salt and pepper.

In a serving bowl, combine the avocado, corn, onions, carrots, celery hearts, cucumbers, mixed greens, and tomatoes. Add the vinaigrette and toss well. Season with salt and pepper, add a splash of sherry vinegar, and sprinkle with Parmesan. Divide onto four plates and serve.

PER SERVING: 170 CALORIES, 11.87G FAT, 13.23G CARBS, 4.34G PROTEIN, 3.46G FIBER, 84MG CALCIUM, 0.70MG IRON, 119MG SODIUM, 52µG FOLATE

apple and celery salad with currants and champagne vinaigrette

This elegant mélange of fruit, vegetables, and almonds can be an outstanding side salad or main course, especially if you add roasted chicken.

Serves 4

1 tablespoon champagne vinegar
1 teaspoon minced shallot
freshly ground black pepper
¼ teaspoon kosher salt
½ teaspoon sugar
⅛ teaspoon Dijon mustard
2 tablespoons canola oil
1 crisp red apple, thinly sliced
½ cup toasted almonds, halved
4 celery stalks, sliced into ½-inch pieces
⅛ cup dried currants
6 cups chopped romaine lettuce hearts

In a small nonreactive bowl, combine the vinegar, shallot, pepper, salt, sugar, and mustard and whisk until blended. Whisk in the oil to combine and set aside.

In a salad bowl, combine the apple, almonds, celery, currants, and romaine leaves. Add the dressing, toss, and serve.

PER SERVING: 219 CALORIES, 15.52G FAT, 17.13G CARBS, 5.28G PROTEIN, 5.56G FIBER, 91MG CALCIUM, 1.80MG IRON, 185MG SODIUM, 117µG FOLATE

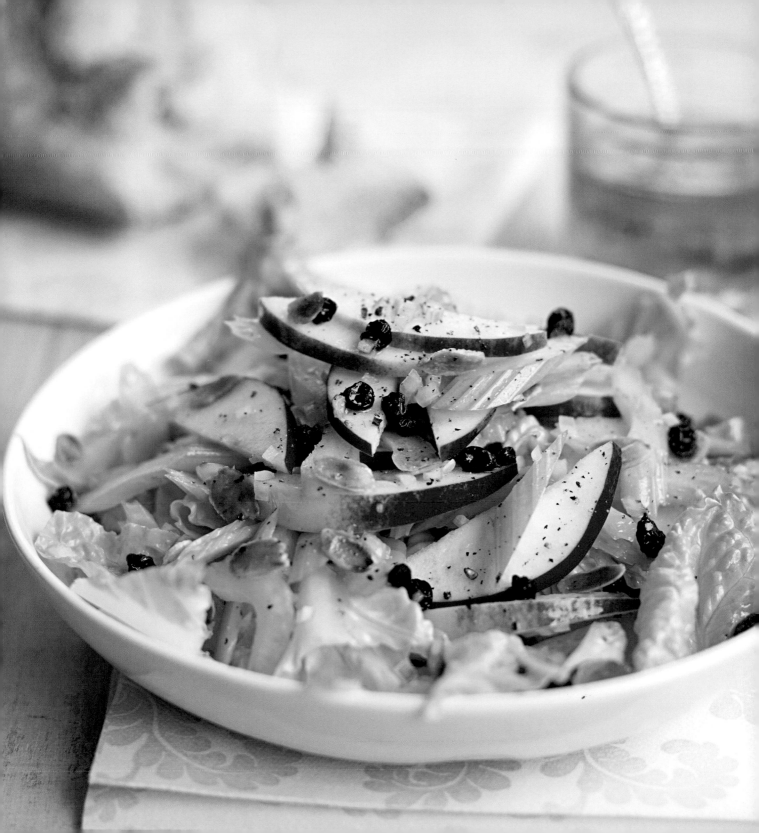

chinese chicken salad

This crunchy, addictive salad with a hot dry-mustard kick pays tribute to Wolfgang Puck's famed Chinois restaurant, as well as to the under-appreciated napa cabbage. Also known as Chinese cabbage, it is low in calories and high in vitamin C and calcium—both of which are very good for your baby and you. Bonus: The dressing's sesame oil is an antioxidant and rich in minerals and vitamins A, B, and E.

Serves 4

¼ cup sliced almonds
2 teaspoons dry Chinese or English (Coleman's) mustard
2 tablespoons seasoned rice vinegar
1½ teaspoons low-sodium soy sauce
1 tablespoon light sesame oil
2 tablespoons canola oil
generous pinch coarse salt
½ teaspoon sugar
freshly ground black pepper
3 cups firmly packed shredded napa cabbage
⅔ cup julienned red bell pepper
1 cup shredded cooked chicken breast

In a small sauté pan over medium heat, toast the almonds, stirring constantly, for 2 to 3 minutes. Remove from heat and set aside.

Combine the mustard, vinegar, soy sauce, sesame and canola oils, salt, sugar, and pepper to taste in a salad bowl and whisk until combined. Add the cabbage, bell pepper, chicken, and almonds, and toss until evenly coated with dressing. Serve.

PER SERVING: 219 CALORIES, 14.00G FAT, 5.46G CARBS, 16.68G PROTEIN, 1.40G FIBER, 57MG CALCIUM, 1.62MG IRON, 276MG SODIUM, 49µG FOLATE

watermelon, arugula, feta, and mint salad

This unexpected combination dances on the palate thanks to the sweetness of watermelon, tartness of lime, saltiness of the feta and olives, and semi-spicy herbaceous character of the arugula. Thanks to tummy-soothing watermelon, it also can be a godsend to the queasy mom. Note: If possible, drain the watermelon cubes by placing them in a colander over a bowl in the refrigerator overnight beforehand.

Serves 4

½ small red onion, sliced thinly and halved (about ¼ cup)
2 tablespoons fresh lime juice
1 tablespoon extra-virgin olive oil
6 kalamata olives, pitted and chopped
1½ cups ripe seedless watermelon, cut into thin triangles
1½ cups loosely packed arugula
¼ cup loosely packed chopped fresh mint
⅓ cup crumbled pasteurized feta cheese

In a serving bowl combine the onion, lime juice, olive oil, and olives and mix until combined and the onions are coated. Let stand for 15 minutes.

Add the watermelon, arugula, mint, and feta. Toss so the dressing coats the lettuce, and serve.

PER SERVING: 104 CALORIES, 6.53G FAT, 9.48G CARBS, 2.91G PROTEIN, 1.27G FIBER, 99MG CALCIUM, 1.16MG IRON, 209MG SODIUM, 28µG FOLATE

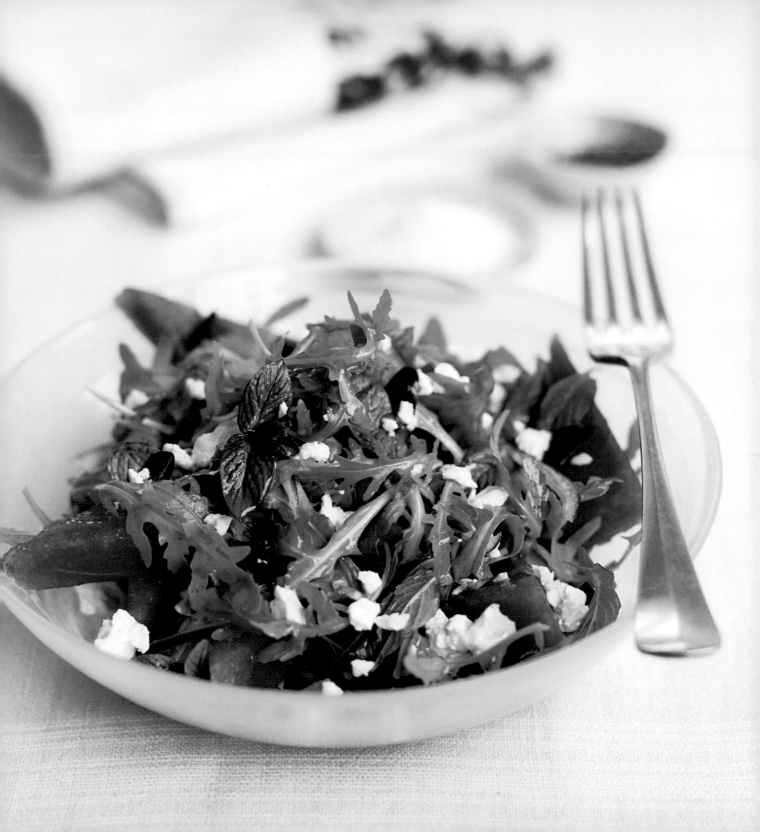

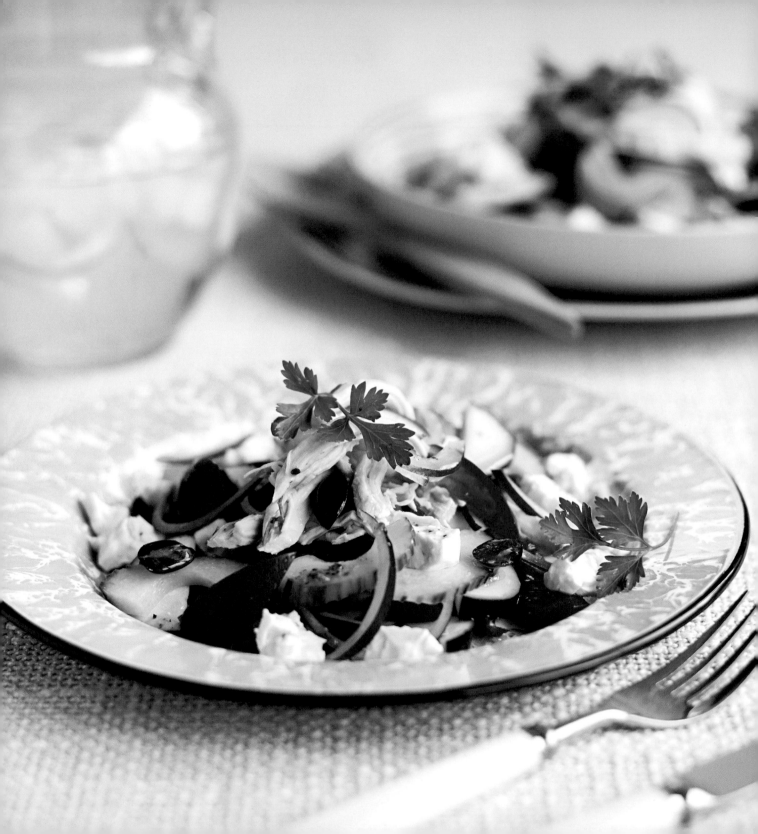

deluxe greek salad

If you love the cool, satisfying goodness that is greek salad, you'll adore this adaptation of "Barefoot Contessa" chef Ina Garten's version. It turns summertime's standby into a hearty side dish or main course and provides much-needed vegetables and protein.

Serves 4

½ teaspoon minced fresh garlic
1 teaspoon dried oregano
¼ teaspoon Dijon mustard
1 tablespoon plus 1 teaspoon red wine vinegar
¼ teaspoon kosher salt
pinch of freshly ground black pepper
3 tablespoons extra-virgin olive oil
1 red bell pepper, seeded and chopped
2 plum or other vine-ripened tomatoes, seeded and
   cut into 1-inch cubes
1 cucumber, seeded and sliced into 1-inch cubes
1 zucchini, peeled and sliced into 1-inch cubes
¾ cup chopped red onion
1 cup cooked chicken, cut into 1-inch cubes
⅓ pound pasteurized feta cheese, crumbled
¼ cup kalamata olives, pitted and chopped
2 sprigs flat-leaf parsely (optional)

In a large mixing bowl, whisk together the garlic, oregano, mustard, vinegar, salt, pepper, and olive oil until combined. Add the bell pepper, tomatoes, cucumber, zucchini, onion, and chicken and gently toss until all the chicken and vegetables are well coated.

Add the feta and olives and toss lightly. Set aside for 30 minutes to allow the flavors to blend before garnishing with parsley and serving.

PER SERVING: 310 CALORIES, 18.74G FAT, 12.83G CARBS, 21.11G PROTEIN, 2.81G FIBER, 236MG CALCIUM, 1.84MG IRON, 696MG SODIUM, 68µG FOLATE

spinach salad with shiitakes, pine nuts, and lemon dressing

Tart, light lemon dressing is the perfect partner for sautéed shiitake mushrooms and flavors of toasted pine nuts. Feel free to add a tablespoon of crumbled feta for visual contrast and creamy deliciousness, or throw in some chopped, cooked bacon for the ultimate decadence.

Serves 4

1 teaspoon olive oil
1 cup sliced fresh shiitake mushrooms
⅛ cup pine nuts
2 tablespoons canola oil
4½ teaspoons fresh lemon juice
⅛ teaspoon kosher salt
pinch of freshly ground black pepper
5 cups spinach leaves, stems removed and loosely packed

Heat the olive oil in a small sauté pan over medium heat until it's hot but not smoking. Add the mushrooms and sauté, stirring frequently, until lightly browned, about 4 minutes. Set aside.

In a small sauté pan over medium heat, add the pine nuts and toast, stirring frequently, about 5 minutes. Let cool.

In a serving bowl, add the canola oil, lemon juice, salt, and pepper, and stir with a fork until completely combined. Add the spinach, mushrooms, and pine nuts and toss. Serve.

PER SERVING: 113 CALORIES, 10.48G FAT, 3.52G CARBS, 2.09G PROTEIN, 1.47G FIBER, 40MG CALCIUM, 1.29MG IRON, 106MG SODIUM, 78µG FOLATE

shaved zucchini and mache salad with lemon and parmesan

Zucchini takes on a whole new—and perhaps surprisingly tasty—personality when served raw, shaved into paper-thin ribbons and drizzled with lemon juice and olive oil. Plus, it's a good source of vitamin C and dietary fiber.

Serves 4

3 medium zucchini, peeled
¼ pound Parmesan, plus more for sprinkling
2 cups baby mache
2 tablespoons extra-virgin olive oil
2 teaspoons lemon juice
salt and freshly ground black pepper
1 tablespoon minced parsley

Using a vegetable peeler, shave the zucchini lengthwise into long ribbons. Then shave the Parmesan into long ribbons. Transfer both to a serving bowl and add the mache.

In a small bowl, whisk together the olive oil and lemon juice and pour it over the vegetables.

Season with salt and pepper, toss lightly, sprinkle with Parmesan and parsley, and serve.

PER SERVING: 197 CALORIES, 13.75G FAT, 6.48G CARBS, 12.21G PROTEIN, 1.82G FIBER, 374MG CALCIUM, 0.99MG IRON, 471MG SODIUM, 55µG FOLATE

roasted beet, orange, and avocado salad

Colorful and loaded with folate, vitamin C, and "good fats," this salad also has wonderful texture thanks to hearty beets, melt-in-your-mouth avocado, and juicy orange slices.

Serves 4

2 medium red beets, tops removed
2 tablespoons canola oil
2 tablespoons balsamic or champagne vinegar
1 tablespoon freshly squeezed orange juice
½ teaspoon kosher salt
freshly ground black pepper
1 ripe orange, peeled
½ ripe but firm avocado, cubed
1 cup mache or baby greens (optional)
¼ cup pasteurized feta cheese, crumbled

Preheat the oven to 400°F. Line a baking dish with foil and place the beets on top. Drizzle with 1 tablespoon canola oil and 1 tablespoon vinegar. Cover tightly with more foil and roast for 45 minutes. Remove from the oven and set aside to cool.

In a small bowl, combine 1 tablespoon oil, 1 tablespoon vinegar, orange juice, salt, and pepper and whisk until combined.

Once the beets have cooled, peel them with a knife, cut them into 1½-inch cubes, and transfer to a serving bowl.

Cut the orange in half and cut out the segments. Add them to the serving bowl along with the avocado and mache, if desired. Drizzle the dressing over, toss to coat, then sprinkle the feta on top and serve.

PER SERVING: 129 CALORIES, 8.72G FAT, 10.53G CARBS, 2.90G PROTEIN, 3.50G FIBER, 74MG CALCIUM, 0.68MG IRON, 430MG SODIUM, 80µG FOLATE

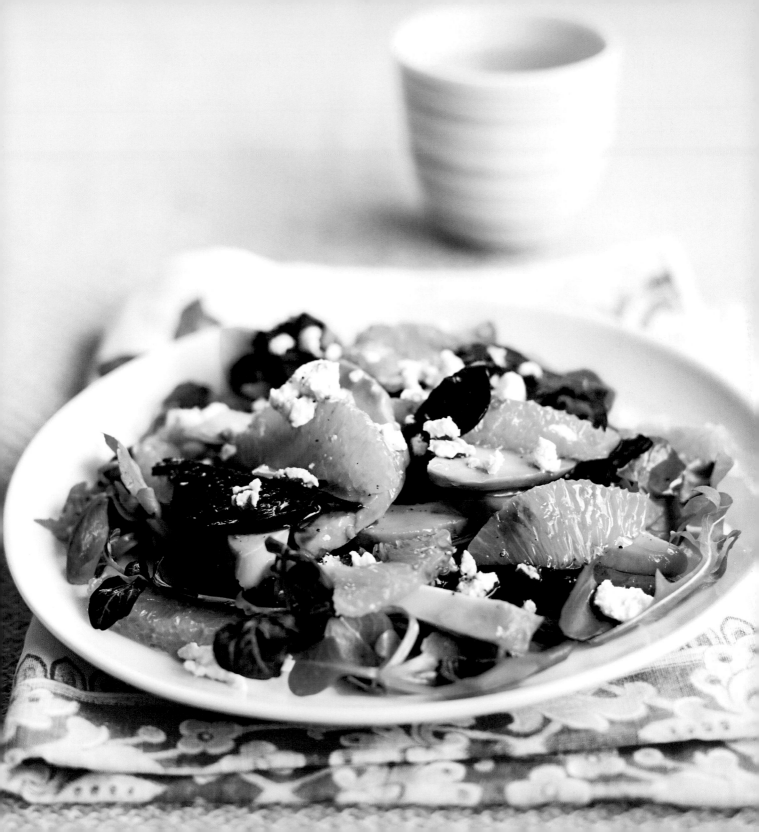

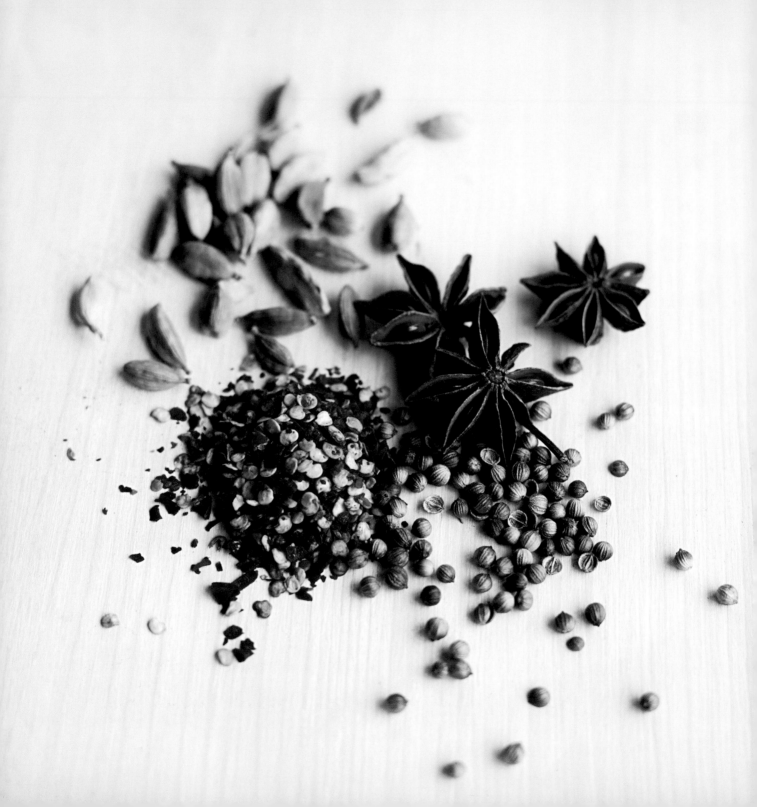

chapter five

main courses

mushroom quinoa risotto

If you're not yet onboard with the recent (and ironically ancient) trend of cooking with quinoa, this guiltlessly decadent recipe is your incentive. Created by cooking instructor, cookbook author, and mother of three Dana Slatkin, it elevates the grain known for its simultaneously soft and crunchy character to gourmet status. The benefits beyond flavor are great: Quinoa is an exceptional source of protein, calcium, iron, and all eight essential amino acids! Tip: Before using quinoa, rinse it once or twice under cold water to remove the slightly bitter residue. Garnish with chives for visual flair.

Serves 4

3 cups mushroom or chicken broth
1 tablespoon plus 2 teaspoons olive oil
2 tablespoons finely chopped shallot
1 teaspoon minced garlic
1½ cups white quinoa, rinsed
½ cup white wine
8 ounces shiitake or white mushrooms, diced
salt and freshly ground black pepper
8 ounces trumpet mushrooms, trimmed and sliced
⅓ cup grated Parmesan, plus extra shavings for serving

In a medium pot, heat the broth over low heat and simmer while you prepare the rest of the dish.

In another medium pot, heat 1 tablespoon olive oil over medium heat. Add the shallot and garlic and sauté until soft and translucent, stirring often to prevent browning. Add the quinoa and cook for a few minutes, stirring, until the grains are coated in oil and fragrant, about 3 minutes.

Add the wine and cook, stirring occasionally, until evaporated. Ladle ½ cup of hot broth into the quinoa, stir, and simmer until the liquid has evaporated, about 3 minutes. Continue the process, adding ½ cup broth at a time, until the quinoa is fully cooked and there is no more broth, about 25 minutes.

Meanwhile, heat the remaining two teaspoons oil in a small sauté pan and cook the shiitake mushrooms until browned. Season with salt and pepper, transfer to a bowl, and set aside. Repeat with the trumpet mushrooms.

Stir the shiitake mushrooms and Parmesan into the risotto. Spoon into 4 serving bowls and top with the trumpet mushrooms. Serve immediately, with additional Parmesan cheese for sprinkling.

PER SERVING: 386 CALORIES, 11.43G FAT, 47.55G CARBS, 17.95G PROTEIN, 5.39G FIBER, 152 MG CALCIUM, 4.12MG IRON, 553MG SODIUM, 141μG FOLATE

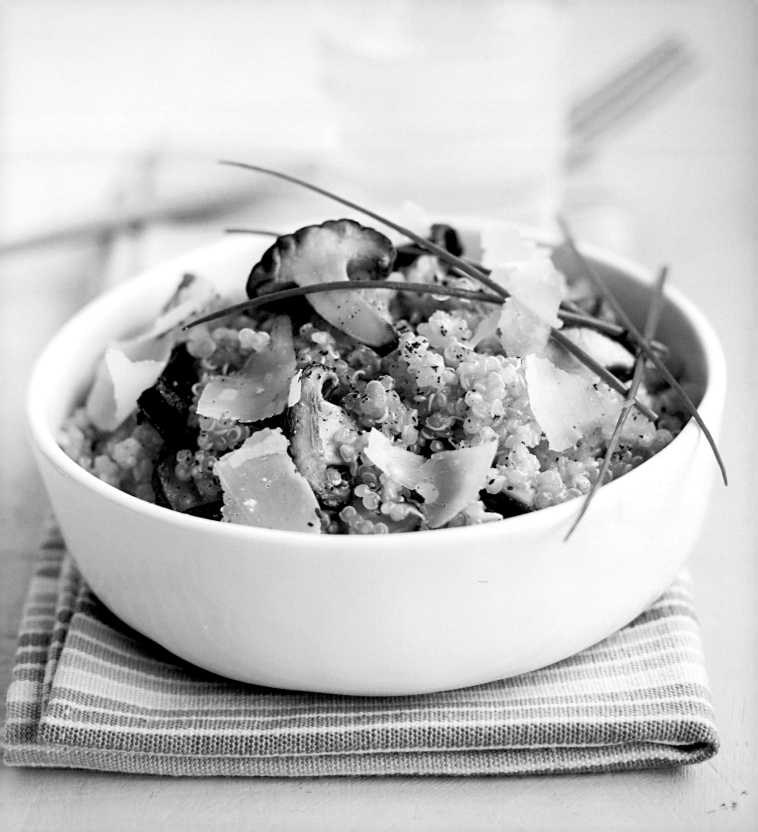

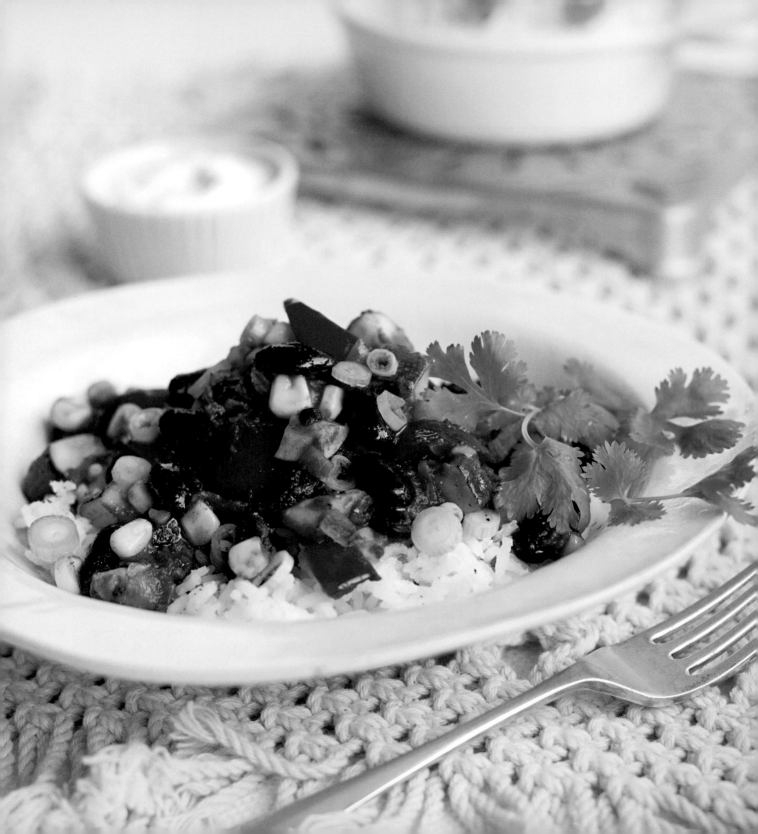

vegetarian chili

Filling and loaded with healthy ingredients, this classic is best garnished with shredded Cheddar, green onions, diced avocado, a dollop of yogurt or sour cream, or fresh minced cilantro. Freeze leftovers for an effortless future meal over a bowl of rice.

Serves 4

2 tablespoons canola oil
2 cups chopped onion
1²/₃ cups coarsely chopped red bell peppers
2 tablespoons chopped garlic
2 tablespoons chili powder
2 teaspoons dried oregano
2 teaspoons ground cumin
¹/₈ teaspoon cayenne
2 (15- to 16-ounce) cans chili beans, drained
½ cup water
2 cups peeled, diced tomatoes with juices
1 cup corn kernels
2 cups cubed fresh zucchini
1 teaspoon kosher salt

Heat the oil in large, heavy pot over medium-high heat. Add the onion, bell peppers, and garlic and sauté until the onions are soft, about 10 minutes. Add the spices and stir to combine. Mix in the beans, water, and tomatoes. Bring to a boil, stirring occasionally, then reduce to medium-low and simmer for 10 minutes. Stir in the corn, zucchini, and salt and simmer for 5 minutes.

Ladle the chili into bowls and serve with any of the embellishments mentioned above.

PER SERVING: 428 CALORIES, 10.15G FAT, 70.76G CARBS, 19.55G PROTEIN, 21.58G FIBER, 195MG CALCIUM, 7.01MG IRON, 1663MG SODIUM, 190µG FOLATE

red snapper with vinaigrette provençal

Red snapper is a fish that is low in mercury, and thus safe to consume in moderation while pregnant. An excellent source of protein, omega-3 fatty acids, and vitamins B6 and B12, it's also a deliciously light partner for the vibrant, tangy flavors of the accompanying vinaigrette.

Serves 4

1 cup finely chopped onion
1 tablespoon minced fresh garlic
2 teaspoons unsalted butter
3 tablespoons sherry vinegar
½ cup seeded and chopped tomato
¹/₃ cup finely chopped red bell pepper
2 tablespoons olive oil
1 tablespoon minced fresh parsley
1 tablespoon finely chopped kalamata olives
kosher salt and freshly ground black pepper
4 (6-ounce) pieces red snapper

In a large skillet, cook the onion, garlic, and butter over medium heat, stirring, until translucent, about 10 minutes.

Add the vinegar and tomato and cook, covered, for 5 minutes. Add the bell pepper and olive oil and cook, stirring, for 2 minutes. Stir in the parsley and olives, season with salt and pepper, transfer to a bowl, and set aside.

Season the fish with salt and pepper, place in the same hot skillet, in batches if necessary, and sauté over medium heat for 3 minutes per side. Transfer the fish to four plates, warm the vinaigrette in the skillet, stirring, and spoon onto each piece of fish. Serve.

PER SERVING: 163 CALORIES, 9.14G FAT, 6.28G CARBS, 12.59G PROTEIN, 1.34G FIBER, 37MG CALCIUM, 0.55MG IRON, 59MG SODIUM, 20µG FOLATE

broiled sake-marinated filet of salmon in shiso broth

Napa Valley's James Beard Award-winning chef Hiro Sone is one of the best chefs in the United States, and this recipe proves the point. Light and easy to prepare, its elegance and complex flavors exude four-star quality—as well as pregnancy essentials like protein and omega-3s from the salmon, and calcium, folic acid, vitamins C and K, iron, and fiber from the spinach. Can't find the exotic herb known as shiso? Skip it and the dish will still elicit a lifelong love affair.

Serves 4

2 tablespoons dry sake
¼ cup soy sauce
2 tablespoon mirin
3 tablespoons granulated sugar
⅛ teaspoon grated peeled ginger
⅛ teaspoon grated garlic
4 (6-ounce) salmon filets, about 1 inch thick (preferably wild salmon)
2 cups chicken broth or water
½ teaspoon rice vinegar
1 cup stemmed and sliced shiitake mushrooms
6 cups fresh spinach
1 green onion, thinly sliced
2 shiso leaves, sliced
1 teaspoon toasted white sesame seeds

Whisk the sake, soy sauce, mirin, sugar, ginger, and garlic in a small mixing bowl. Reserve 3 tablespoons of the marinade. Marinate the salmon, covered and refrigerated, for at least 3 hours or overnight, in the remaining marinade.

Preheat the broiler or oven to 500°F. Rinse the marinade off the salmon and pat dry. Place the salmon on a sauté pan or baking sheet, place under the broiler, and cook until the surface turns a nice mahogany color, about 10 minutes.

Meanwhile, combine the broth, reserved sake marinade, vinegar, and mushrooms in a medium saucepan and bring to a boil. Add the spinach and green onion and bring to a boil.

Divide the broth and vegetables into 4 serving bowls. Sprinkle with the shiso. Place one salmon filet in the middle of each bowl, sprinkle with the sesame seeds, and serve.

PER SERVING: 175 CALORIES, 3.68G FAT, 20.94G CARBS, 13.36G PROTEIN, 2.82G FIBER, 88MG CALCIUM, 2.97MG IRON, 1276MG SODIUM, 126µG FOLATE

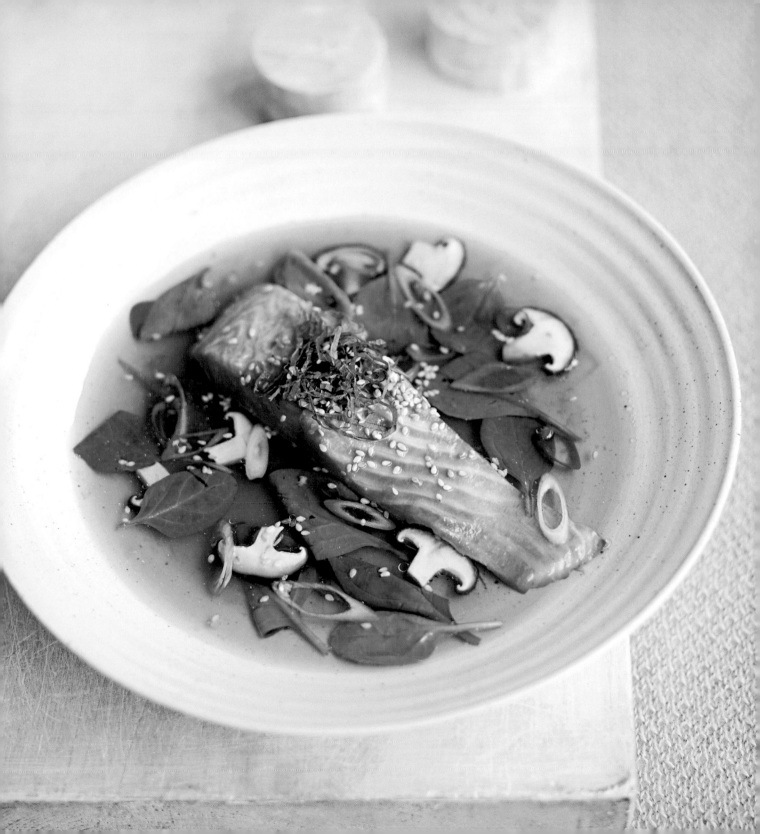

sautéed salmon with green beans, tomatoes, and sherry vinaigrette

Salmon is one of the best types of fish you can eat while pregnant due to its high amount of protein and omega-3 fatty acids, the latter of which are essential for a baby's brain development. This elegant preparation is big on flavor and low on effort and calories. What else could a hungry pregnant woman ask for—except, perhaps, someone else to prepare it for her.

Serves 4

4 tablespoons plus 2 teaspoons extra-virgin olive oil
2 tablespoons sherry vinegar
1½ teaspoons minced shallot
1 teaspoon kosher salt
20 cherry or grape tomatoes, halved
4 cups green beans, ends trimmed
4 (4-ounce) salmon fillets (preferably wild salmon)

Combine 4 tablespoons olive oil, the sherry vinegar, shallot, and salt in a small mixing bowl. Stir to combine. Add the tomatoes, stir to coat, and set aside.

Bring a large pot of water to a boil and blanch the green beans until crisp but not raw, about 3 minutes. Quickly transfer the beans to a bowl of ice water to cool. Drain.

Heat the remaining 2 teaspoons of oil in large skillet over medium-high heat. Generously sprinkle the salmon with salt and pepper then cook it in the skillet, in batches if necessary, about 4 minutes per side, or until brown and crisp on the outside and just cooked through on the inside. Transfer to plates and keep warm.

Add the tomatoes, vinaigrette, and green beans to the hot skillet and warm for 2 to 3 minutes, or until the tomatoes begin to soften. Pour over the salmon and serve.

PER SERVING: 380 CALORIES, 24.05G FAT, 11.41G CARBS, 26.94G PROTEIN, 4.76G FIBER, 56MG CALCIUM, 2.05MG IRON, 646MG SODIUM, 58µG FOLATE

miso-marinated black cod with japanese-style steamed spinach and edamame

Elegant enough to serve to company and easy enough to prepare for a midweek meal, this spin on famed Japanese chef Nobu Matsuhisa's rich miso-marinated black cod is a winning combination of dense and lightly flavored fish coated with a sweet and savory miso glaze, plus iron-rich (and wholly addictive) steamed spinach. The edamame adds whimsically decorative nibbles to the dish, but can be easily skipped, if desired.

Serves 4

2 tablespoons sake
2 tablespoons mirin
½ cup yellow miso paste
¼ cup plus 2 tablespoons sugar
4 (⅓-pound) black cod fillets
12 ounces fresh baby spinach
3 tablespoons white sesame seeds
2½ tablespoons soy sauce
¼ cup cooked shucked edamame beans

In a medium saucepan, bring the saké and the mirin to a boil over high heat. Boil for 20 seconds to evaporate the alcohol. Remove from the heat, add the miso paste and ¼ cup sugar and stir until combined. Let cool.

Place the fish in a single layer in a container with a tight-sealing cover. Generously coat each piece of cod with the miso mixture, cover, and refrigerate overnight or up to 30 hours.

Preheat the broiler.

Wipe off, but don't rinse, all of the miso sauce from the fish. Transfer to a broiler pan or baking sheet and broil until the fish caramelizes to a light brown. Turn off the broiler and turn the oven to 400°F. Bake for 10 to 15 minutes.

Fill a large pot with an inch of water fitted with a steamer. Bring the water to a boil, place the spinach in the steamer, in batches if necessary, cover, and steam the spinach for 2 minutes or until wilted. Remove the spinach, drain, and cool. Squeeze any excess water out of the spinach, chop coarsely, and set aside.

Toast the sesame seeds in a dry frying pan over high heat, about 2 minutes or until light brown. Using a coffee grinder or food processor, grind the seeds. Add the remaining 2 tablespoons sugar and grind until the mixture becomes a paste. Add the soy sauce and blend.

In a bowl, combine the spinach and sesame seed dressing thoroughly. Serve alongside the cod. Garnish with the edamame beans.

PER SERVING: 168 CALORIES, 2.55G FAT, 8.82 CARBS, 26.24G PROTEIN, 3.04G FIBER, 136MG CALCIUM, 3.66MG IRON, 944MG SODIUM, 201µG FOLATE

tacolicious fish tacos

If anyone knows how to do tacos right, it's San Francisco's
Tacolicious. The restaurant focuses squarely on exciting
ingredients expertly prepared and neatly tucked into warm
tortillas. This recipe—a home cook–friendly version of one of their
specials—underscores their expertise. A mélange of light, spice-
spiked fish, tangy Greek yogurt, and lime-kissed slaw, it can be
devoured with the confidence that your meal is not only delicious
but also a good source of protein and vitamins C, B6, B12, and K.

Serves 4

2 teaspoons ground ancho chile powder
1 teaspoon ground chipotle chile powder
  or chili powder
1 teaspoon garlic powder
1 teaspoon dried oregano
1½ teaspoons kosher salt
½ cup plain Greek yogurt, drained
1 teaspoon ground cumin
6 teaspoons fresh lime juice
2 cups shredded cabbage
2 to 3 radishes, thinly sliced
¼ cup chopped cilantro
1 tablespoon olive oil
1 pound cod filet, cut in 2-inch pieces
8 (5- to 6-inch) corn or flour tortillas
1 avocado, chopped

In a small bowl, mix the ancho and chipotle chile powders, garlic powder,
oregano, and ½ teaspoon salt. Season the fish with a light sprinkle of the
"ancho recado" spices and set aside.

In a nonreactive bowl, mix the yogurt, cumin, 2 teaspoons lime juice, and
½ teaspoon salt, and refrigerate. In another nonreactive bowl, mix the shredded
cabbage, sliced radishes, cilantro, 4 teaspoons lime juice and set aside.

Heat the olive oil in a cast-iron or nonstick skillet and cook the fish about
2 to 3 minutes per side.

Warm the tortillas by wrapping them in foil and heating them in a warm oven.
To assemble, place some avocado and a piece of fish in the center of each
tortilla, and top with 1 tablespoon of the yogurt mix and some of the cabbage-
radish slaw.

PER SERVING: 326 CALORIES, 12.17G FAT, 28.88G CARBS, 26.23G PROTEIN, 7.85G FIBER, 149MG CALCIUM,
2.22MG IRON, 1006MG SODIUM, 76μG FOLATE

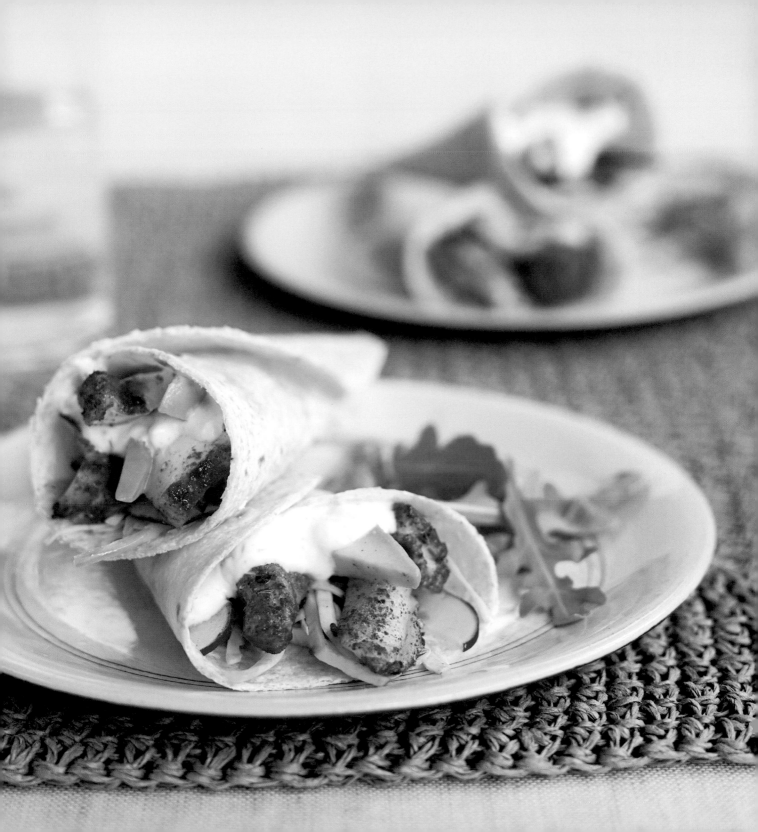

curried scallops with smoky lentils

These lentils, inspired by a recipe in the divine *Summertime Anytime Cookbook*, are an excellent source of dietary fiber and iron. Scallops are superb providers of protein, vitamin B12, phosphorus, and selenium. Married with bacon and curry powder, they are a direct route to dinnertime divinity. Tip: To mince the bacon, partially freeze and cut it before it thaws.

Serves 4

2 strips thick-cut nitrate-free bacon, minced
¾ cup French or black lentils
¼ cup minced shallot
⅓ cup diced carrot
2 tablespoons diced celery
1¼ cups low-sodium chicken broth
kosher salt and freshly ground black pepper
2 tablespoons curry powder
12 large sea scallops
1 tablespoon canola oil

In a small saucepan over medium heat, cook the bacon just until it begins to brown. Add the lentils, shallot, carrot, and celery. Stir to coat with the bacon grease and cook for about 2 minutes. Add the chicken broth, a generous pinch of salt, and black pepper to taste, and simmer, uncovered and stirring occasionally, until the lentils are soft, about 30 minutes.

Meanwhile, place the curry powder on a plate with generous pinches of salt and pepper and dredge the scallops in the curry mixture; set aside.

Place the canola oil into a large sauté pan and heat until hot but not smoking. Brown the scallops on each side for 2 to 3 minutes.

To serve, divide the cooked lentils on 4 dinner plates and top each plate with 3 curried scallops.

PER SERVING: 252 CALORIES, 6.04G FAT, 28.47G CARBS, 20.63G PROTEIN, 12.48G FIBER, 59MG CALCIUM, 4.20MG IRON, 277MG SODIUM, 192µG FOLATE

fast and fabulous paella

Napa Valley's Zuzu restaurant is beloved for its paella. This adaptation, based on original chef Charles Weber's exceptional and far more complicated recipe, pays tribute to the flavor minus the labor. It's also got good protein plus vitamin C from the bell pepper. Tips: Ask your grocer to halve the baby back ribs crosswise so they are bite-size when you cook and serve them. Or swap them for slices of chicken breast if you like. And don't forget the safe-shellfish rule of thumb: If its shell doesn't open up during cooking, don't eat it because it could make you sick. You can also skip the shellfish and the dish will still deliver.

Serves 4

1½ cups chicken broth
½ cup tomato juice
¼ cup chopped yellow onion
½ cup seeded and chopped red bell pepper
3 cloves fresh garlic
1 bay leaf
pinch of saffron
1 pound baby back ribs, halved
¼ teaspoon kosher salt
2 teaspoons olive oil
¾ cup paella rice (available at gourmet
   food stores)
½ cup frozen green peas
¼ cup hard chorizo
8 raw shrimp, peeled
8 clams
8 mussels

In a medium pot over medium heat, combine the chicken broth, vegetable juice, onion, bell pepper, 2 garlic cloves, bay leaf, and saffron and bring to a boil. Slice the ribs into individual riblets and add them to the broth. Reduce to a simmer, and cook for 20 minutes. Stir in the salt, taste, add more if needed, and let cool. Discard the bay leaf and remove and set aside the ribs.

Transfer the liquid to a blender and blend until combined.

Preheat the oven to 450°F. Slice the remaining garlic clove thinly. Heat the olive oil in a large ovenproof sauté pan over medium heat. Add the sliced garlic and saute for 2 minutes. Add the paella rice, stir to coat, and scatter evenly around the bottom of the pan.

Arrange the ribs, in one layer, evenly on top of the rice. Scatter the peas and chorizo around the ribs, then add the liquid from the blender. Cook in the upper half of the oven for 15 minutes.

Without stirring the paella, take a test bite from the side of the pan. If there isn't moisture surrounding the rice, add a few tablespoons of water. Add the shrimp, clams, and mussels evenly and cook for 10 more minutes, or until the rice has a bit of crunch at the edges but is not undercooked. Remove and serve.

PER SERVING: 310 CALORIES, 18.74G FAT, 12.83G CARBS, 21.11G PROTEIN, 2.81G FIBER, 89MG CALCIUM, 9.25MG IRON, 696MG SODIUM, 131µG FOLATE

beef and vegetable skewers

Serve these solo or with rice, and don't forget to cook your meat until it's at least medium. If you don't have a grill, use the broiler instead; just don't put the skewers too close to the flame or they'll burn.

Seves 4

1 tablespoon white vinegar
2 tablespoons canola oil
3 cloves garlic, thinly sliced
2 tablespoons plus 1 teaspoon low-sodium soy sauce
2 tablespoons brown sugar
1 pound beef sirloin, cut into 1½-inch cubes (about 24 pieces)
8 wooden skewers
8 white mushrooms, halved
1 red bell pepper, seeded and cut into 2½-inch pieces
1 zucchini, cut into 1-inch-thick rounds
1 Japanese eggplant, cut into 1-inch-thick rounds

In a resealable bag, combine the vinegar, oil, garlic, soy sauce, and brown sugar. Add the beef and marinate, refrigerated, for 2 hours or overnight.

Preheat the grill or broiler. Soak the skewers in water.

To assemble the skewers, slide a cube of meat, a half mushroom, a piece of red bell pepper, another cube of meat, a zucchini slice, an eggplant slice, and another cube of meat onto a skewer. Baste with the marinade. Repeat with all the skewers.

Gently place the skewers on the grill, and cook for 8 minutes or until the meat is just cooked, flipping once. Serve.

PER SERVING: 205 CALORIES, 4.10G FAT, 12.43G CARBS, 28.43G PROTEIN, 6.18G FIBER, 50MG CALCIUM, 2.63MG IRON, 73MG SODIUM, 77µG FOLATE

rosemary and garlic chicken under a brick

This moist, rustic, and simple recipe delivers big flavor (and protein) with little guilt, especially if you discard the chicken skin after cooking. Served with blanched veggies tossed in pan juices, this is a perfect midweek meal.

Serves 4

2 large carrots, peeled and cut into ½-inch rounds
2 medium zucchini, cut in half lengthwise and sliced
2 (8-ounce) skin-on boneless chicken breasts
1 tablespoon minced fresh rosemary
2 teaspoons minced fresh garlic
1 teaspoon kosher salt, plus more as needed
2 teaspoons olive oil

Bring a large pot of water to a boil, add the carrots, and cook for 4 minutes. Add the zucchini, cook for 2 more minutes, then drain and set aside. Meanwhile, rinse and pat dry the chicken.

Mix together the rosemary, garlic, and 1 teaspoon salt and rub it all over the chicken. In a large sauté pan, heat the oil over medium-high heat. Add the chicken, skin-side up. Place a cast-iron or other heavy pan or brick that can fit into the pan on top of the chicken, and cook for 6 minutes. Flip the chicken so it's skin-side down, put the pan or brick back on top, and cook for 6 more minutes. Remove and let rest.

Add the carrots, zucchini, and 1 teaspoon water to the pan and deglaze while heating and coating the vegetables with the pan juices. Season with salt.

Slice the chicken, divide among 4 plates, and serve with the zucchini and carrots.

PER SERVING: 247 CALORIES, 11.97G FAT, 7.28G CARBS, 25.27G PROTEIN, 2.18G FIBER, 42MG CALCIUM, 1.36MG IRON, 687MG SODIUM, 39µG FOLATE

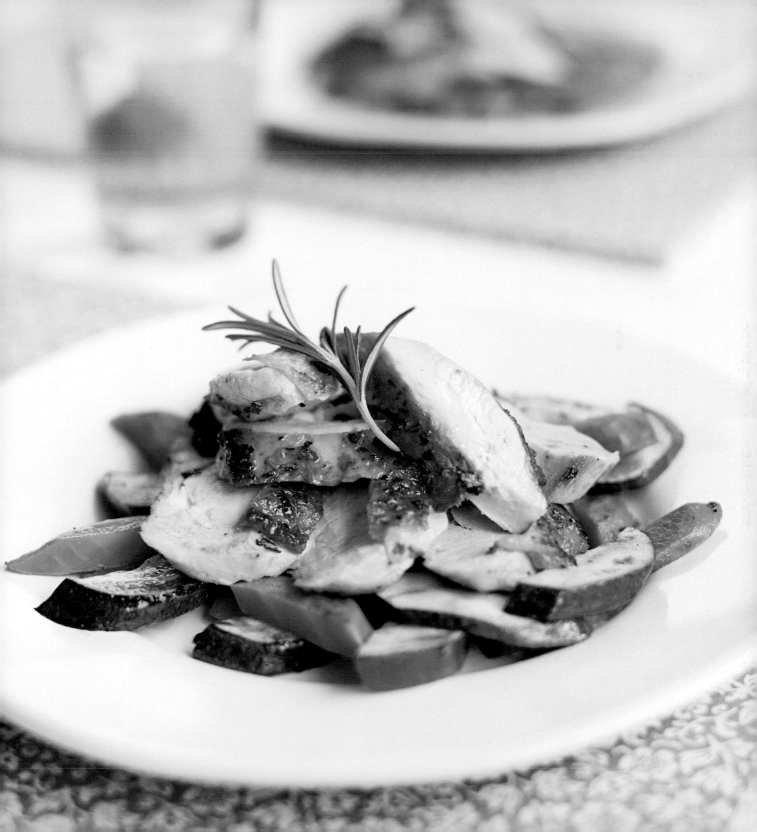

grilled herb chicken

Here, the fresh, vibrant flavors of the garden brighten up the everyday chicken breast without adding on too much in the way of unnecessary calories. Serve it with Grilled Vegetables (page 116), over Lime Rice with Black Beans and Cilantro (page 120), or sliced and layered in a sandwich with lettuce, tomato, mustard, and avocado. Don't have a grill? Bake the chicken at 350°F for 20 to 30 minutes, until cooked through.

Serves 4

¼ onion
2 tablespoons canola oil
3 tablespoons freshly squeezed
  lemon juice
1 teaspoon dried oregano
1 teaspoon chopped fresh rosemary
2 fresh sage leaves, chopped
2 heaping tablespoons minced fresh
  parsley leaves
1 teaspoon fresh thyme leaves
½ clove garlic, minced
¾ teaspoon kosher salt
pinch freshly ground black pepper
4 (6-ounce) boneless, skinless
  chicken breasts

Finely grate the onion over a plate. Transfer the grated onion and its juice into a blender. Add the oil, lemon juice, oregano, rosemary, sage, parsley, thyme, garlic, salt, and pepper and blend until combined.

Transfer to a sauté pan and simmer for 5 minutes over moderate heat. Let cool. Cover the chicken pieces with the herb mixture and place in a nonreactive container just large enough to fit. Marinate for at least 10 minutes or up to 2 hours, refrigerated.

Preheat the grill. Place the chicken on the grill away from direct flame, baste with the marinade, and grill for 4 to 6 minutes. Flip the chicken, baste again, and cook for 4 to 6 minutes, or until cooked through. Let the chicken rest for 5 to 10 minutes and then cut into 1/2-inch slices.

Serve hot or at room temperature.

PER SERVING: 254 CALORIES, 8.20G FAT, 2.37G CARBS, 39.56G PROTEIN, 0.55G FIBER, 35MG CALCIUM, 1.68MG IRON, 547MG SODIUM, 13μG FOLATE

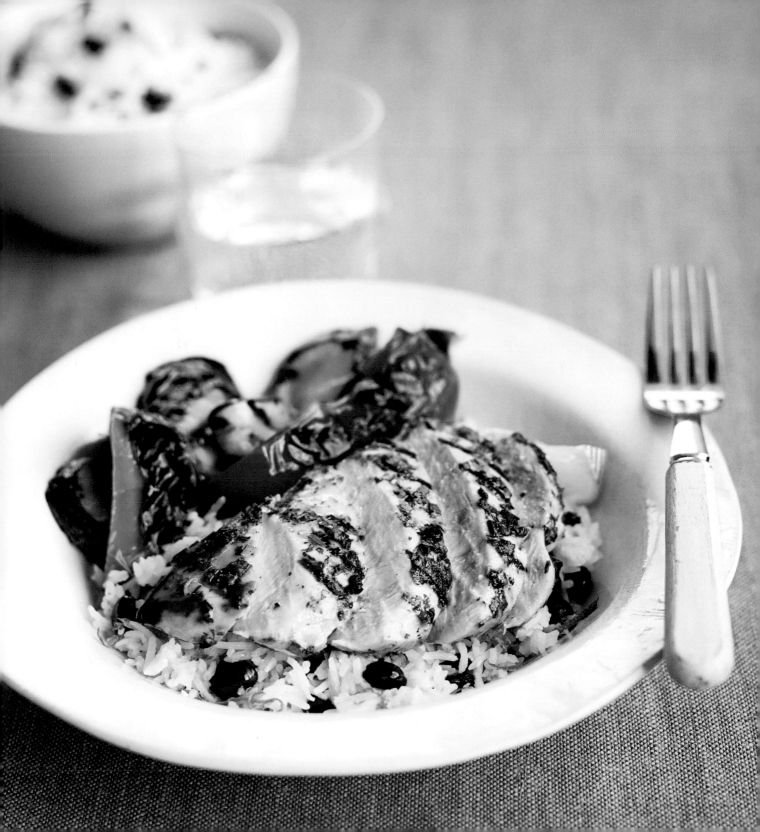

maple-glazed pork chops with mashed sweet potatoes

Sweet tooths needn't suffer through healthy meals in anticipation of dessert with this dish. Here, protein-rich pork and pureed sweet potatoes (an incredible source of fiber, vitamin B6, and potassium) taste downright decadent thanks to their tangy maple glaze.

Seves 4

4 tablespoons pure maple syrup
2 tablespoons Dijon mustard
2 teaspoons apple cider vinegar
4 (5- to 6-ounce) boneless pork chops,
   (about 1 inch thick)
2 medium sweet potatoes, peeled
   and cut into 1½-inch cubes
½ onion (optional)
½ cup low-fat milk
¾ teaspoon kosher salt
freshly ground black pepper
1 teaspoon canola oil

In a mixing bowl, mix the maple syrup, mustard, and vinegar until thoroughly combined. Transfer the mixture to a large sealable bag, add the pork chops and make sure they are well coated. Marinate in the refrigerator for at least 2 hours or overnight.

Preheat the oven to 375°F.

Bring a large pot of salted water to a boil. Add the potatoes and onion and cook until tender, about 15 minutes. Discard the onion, drain the potatoes in a strainer, and leave them until they are dry. Transfer the potatoes to a food processor and puree. Add the milk, salt, and pepper to taste; keep warm.

In a sauté pan, heat the oil until hot but not smoking. Remove the pork chops from the marinade, allowing the excess to drip back into the bag; reserve the marinade. Brown the chops, about 2 minutes per side, then transfer them to a baking pan. Spoon 1 teaspoon marinade over each chop and bake for 10 to 12 minutes or until just cooked through.

Meanwhile, transfer the reserved marinade to a small saucepan and reduce over low heat until thick, about 7 minutes; keep warm. To serve, divide the pureed sweet potatoes onto each dinner plate. Add a pork chop and drizzle with the maple sauce.

PER SERVING: 305 CALORIES, 5.30G FAT, 28.68G CARBS, 35.78G PROTEIN, 2.39G FIBER, 93MG CALCIUM, 1.50MG IRON, 915MG SODIUM, 8µG FOLATE

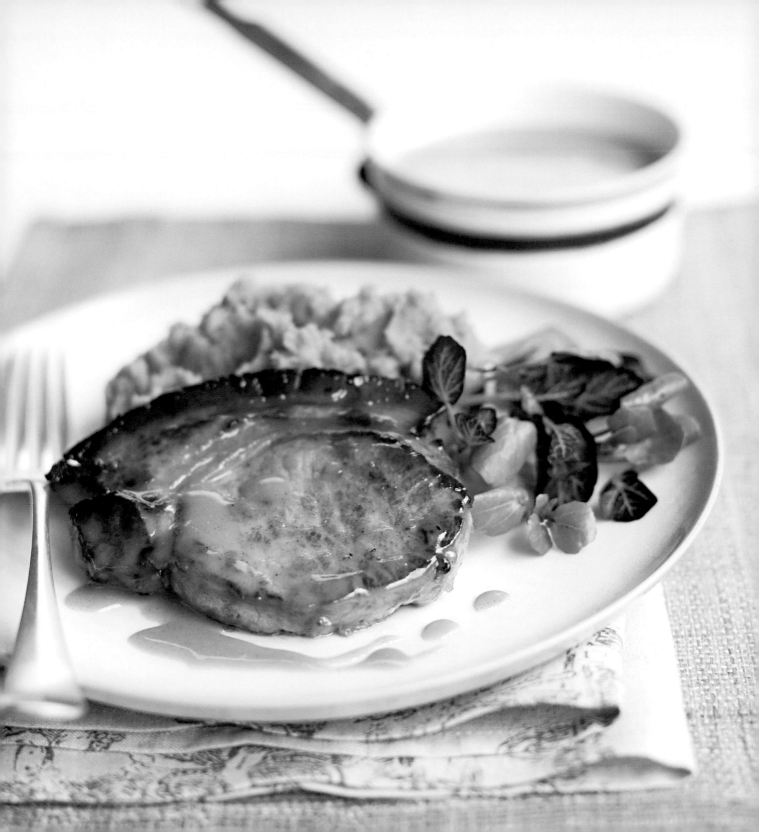

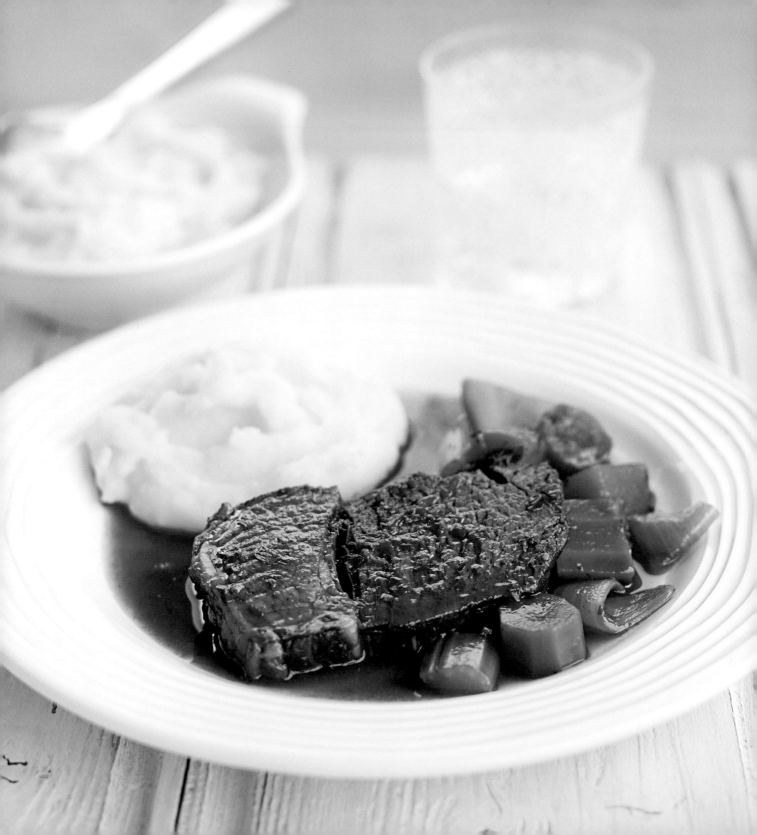

comforting pot roast

What's not to love about throwing a bunch of ingredients in a pot, putting it on the stove, and returning just in time to devour tender chunks of beef slathered in a rich yet surprisingly wholesome sauce that's stocked with veggies? Adapted from a family recipe shared by talented chef Brett McKee of Oak Steakhouse in Charleston, South Carolina, this vivacious pot roast has staying power, because, as McKee promises, good pot roast gets better and more flavorful as leftovers. Serve it solo or with mashed potatoes, and no need to worry about the alcohol content of the included red wine; it evaporates during cooking.

Serves 4

2 teaspoons olive oil
1½-pound beef roast (top or
   bottom round)
salt and freshly ground black pepper
2 celery stalks, roughly diced
2 large carrots, roughly diced
½ large onion, roughly diced
1 yellow beet, roughly diced
1 parsnip, roughly diced
1 clove garlic, peeled
1½ teaspoons tomato paste
¾ cup red wine
3 cups beef broth
2 tablespoons chopped fresh parsley
1 teaspoon chopped fresh thyme

In a Dutch oven or large pot with a lid, heat the olive oil until hot but not smoking. Season the beef with salt and pepper, place it in the hot olive oil, and brown it on all sides. Remove and set aside.

Add the celery, carrots, onion, beet, and parsnip to the pot and cook until they begin to brown. Add the garlic and tomato paste, cook for 1 to 3 minutes, then add the wine and bring to a boil. Boil for 2 minutes, then add the beef broth, parsley, thyme, and beef. Reduce the heat to low and simmer, covered, for 3 hours.

Remove the lid and continue cooking for 30 minutes while the sauce reduces. Season with salt and pepper if desired.

To serve, place a ¾-inch slice of the roast on a plate and ladle the vegetables and sauce over the meat.

PER SERVING: 380 CALORIES, 8.97G FAT, 17.25G CARBS, 44.92G PROTEIN, 4.04G FIBER, 94MG CALCIUM, 5.40MG IRON, 1376MG SODIUM, 96µG FOLATE

pasta bolognese

A shortcut to the satisfying Bolognese-style meat sauce in Marcella Hazan's *The Classic Italian Cookbook,* this recipe is a great midweek meal—especially since kids love it, too. You can dive into a big bowl with reassurance that it's providing necessary protein. Use whole-wheat pasta and you've added fiber to the mix.

Serves 4

1 tablespoon olive oil
½ pound extra-lean ground beef (less than 9% fat)
½ cup dry white wine
¼ cup milk
1 cup marinara sauce
½ teaspoon kosher salt
pinch nutmeg
8 ounces spaghetti
freshly grated Parmesan, for serving (optional)

Heat the oil in a medium saucepan over medium heat. Add the beef and stir frequently to break it up, until it's no longer pink, about 5 minutes. Add the wine, increase the heat to medium-high, and cook until the wine has evaporated, stirring occasionally, about 10 minutes. Add the milk and again simmer until evaporated, stirring occasionally, about 5 minutes. Add the marinara sauce, salt, and nutmeg, simmer for 5 minutes, and keep warm.

Bring a large pot of salted water to a boil and cook the spaghetti, following the directions on the package, until barely al dente. Drain and transfer to four serving bowls. Top each with a quarter of the sauce and serve with grated Parmesan, if desired.

PER SERVING: 428 CALORIES, 10.87G FAT, 52.66G CARBS, 20.39G PROTEIN, 3.50G FIBER, 52MG CALCIUM, 3.71MG IRON, 146µG FOLATE

korean beef broccoli

The Korean-style marinade and super-thin slicing make this dish's meat tender and flavorful, even when well done. For best results, slice the beef when it's partially frozen and stir-fry until just cooked through. If you're craving spicy food, add some red pepper flakes to the pan.

Serves 4

1 pound beef top sirloin or rib-eye, thinly sliced
1 heaping tablespoon minced garlic
2 tablespoons grated onion
3 tablespoons soy sauce
1 tablespoon sugar
1 tablespoon honey
1 tablespoon sesame oil
1 tablespoon sesame seeds, plus more for garnish
pinch freshly ground black pepper
4 cups broccoli florets, halved lengthwise
1 scallion, sliced into thin strips, for garnish

In a large resealable plastic bag, combine the beef, garlic, onion, soy sauce, sugar, honey, sesame oil, sesame seeds, and pepper. Seal, and refrigerate for 2 to 3 hours.

Steam or boil the broccoli until cooked but still firm. Set aside to cool.

Heat a sauté pan over medium-high heat. Add the beef cubes, shaking off any marinade, and cook, stirring frequently, for 3 to 6 minutes, or until done. Add the broccoli during the last two minutes of cooking, to heat and coat with the cooking juices. If the pan gets too dry, add a little water. Garnish with sliced scallions and serve.

PER SERVING: 247 CALORIES, 9.39G FAT, 10.64G CARBS, 28.16G PROTEIN, 0.19G FIBER, 70MG CALCIUM, 2.81MG IRON, 649MG SODIUM, 67µG FOLATE

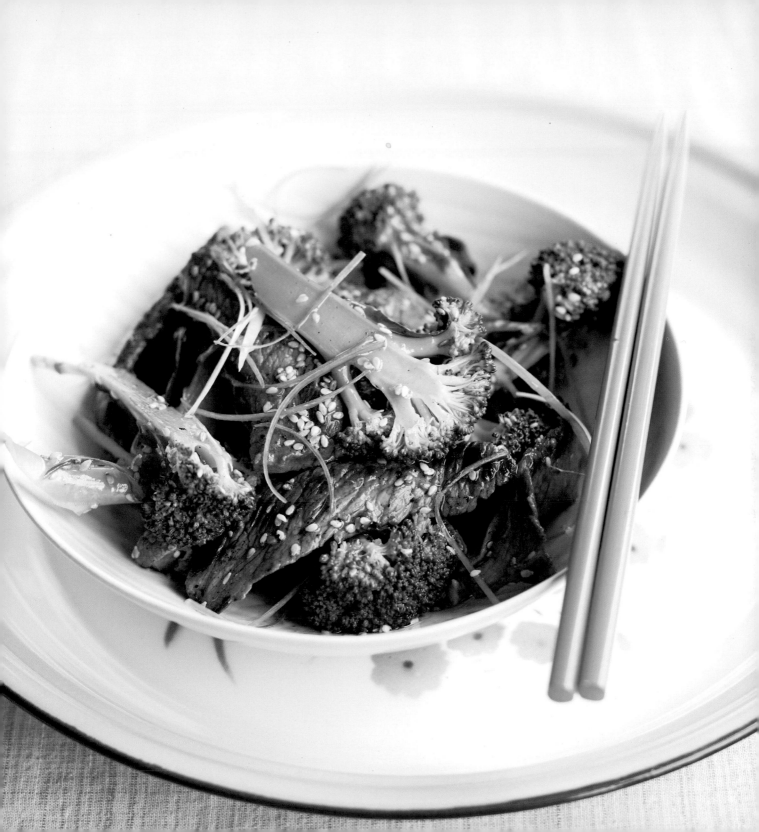

pistachio- and herb-crusted rack of lamb with roasted asparagus and rosemary potatoes

This nut-crusted riff on famed British chef Gordon Ramsey's herb crusted rack of lamb featured on his BBC show "The F Word" is elegant enough to serve on special occasions and easy enough to prepare on weeknights. Along with style, it imparts you ample protein from the lamb and fiber from the nuts.

4 small red potatoes, halved
5 teaspoons extra-virgin olive oil
2 teaspoons chopped fresh rosemary
kosher salt and freshly ground
   black pepper
¾ pounds asparagus, stems trimmed
½ cup minced fresh parsley
1 teaspoon chopped fresh thyme
⅓ cup dry-roasted pistachios
2 (6-rib) frenched racks of lamb
   (each rack ¾ of a pound),
   trimmed of all but a thin layer of fat
1 tablespoon Dijon mustard

Preheat the oven to 400°F.

In a wide bowl, toss the cut potatoes in 2 teaspoons olive oil and 1 teaspoon chopped rosemary to coat. Season with salt and pepper and transfer, cut-side down, in a single layer to a rimmed baking sheet. Roll the asparagus in the same wide bowl, coating with the remaining oil, and set aside. Roast the potatoes for 35 minutes. Add the asparagus in a single layer and roast the potatoes and asparagus for 10 more minutes, then keep warm.

Meanwhile, blend the parsley, thyme, and remaining 1 teaspoon rosemary in a blender or food processor until minced. Add the pistachios and blend or process until minced. Add 1 teaspoon of olive oil and pulse until combined. Set aside.

Season the lamb with salt and pepper. Heat 2 teaspoons olive oil in a large sauté pan over medium-high. Sear the meat one rack at a time by cooking the ribs until brown, turning once, about 5 minutes. Transfer the lamb to a large roasting pan, meat-side up, and coat them with the Dijon mustard.

Gently press the pistachio mixture onto the meaty portion of the rack (not the bones). Roast the lamb until a thermometer inserted diagonally 2 inches into its center (do not touch the bone) registers 155°F (for medium), 20 to 25 minutes. Transfer to a cutting board.

Let stand 10 minutes, then gently cut the meat into individual ribs. Serve with the potatoes and asparagus.

PER SERVING: 571 CALORIES, 29.27G FAT, 34.01G CARBS, 39.86G PROTEIN, 6.20G FIBER, 81MG CALCIUM, 6.95MG IRON, 473MG SODIUM, 123µG FOLATE

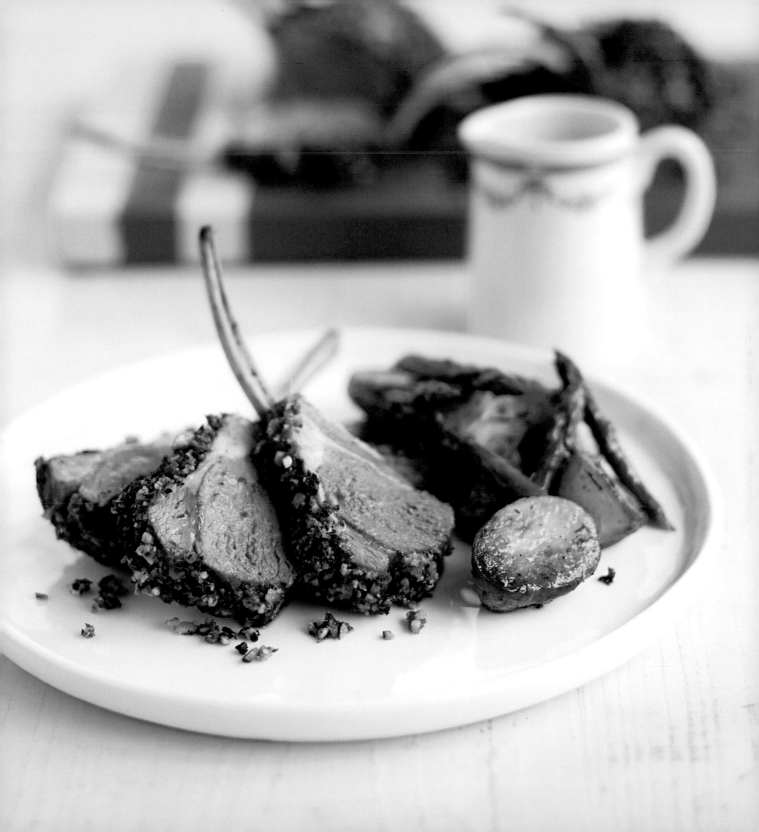

bucatini with fresh fava beans and guanciale

World-class flavor plus folate, dietary fiber, and protein are yours with this recipe from James Beard Award-winning chef Craig Stoll. The owner of San Francisco's famed Delfina is known for transforming rustic, straightforward Italian cooking into astonishingly good food. Part of his secret is fresh, seasonal ingredients, especially in this case, as the dish is best made in late spring or early summer when fava beans are starchier. Incidentally, guanciale is cured hog jowl, similar in texture and flavor to pancetta, which can be substituted in this recipe.

Serves 4–6

½ cup guanciale or pancetta, (nitrate-free),
   diced into ½-inch pieces
2 tablespoons extra-virgin olive oil
2 peeled cloves garlic
kosher salt and freshly ground black pepper
1 tablespoon chopped Italian parsley
5 pounds fava beans, shucked, blanched,
   and peeled (about 2 cups)
1 cup water
1 pound bucatini
3 tablespoons Parmigiano-Reggiano
1 tablespoon extra-virgin olive oil
freshly grated Pecorino-Romano

Add the diced guanciale and olive oil to a heavy-bottomed sauté pan. Slowly render the fat from the guanciale until golden and crispy.

Using the side of a chef's knife, smash the garlic and smear it against the cutting board with a pinch of kosher salt. Add the smashed garlic to the pan and reduce the heat. Cook slowly until the garlic dissolves into the fat but does not brown. Add the parsley, fry briefly, then add the fava beans and water. Season with salt and pepper. Bring to a boil and then reduce to a simmer. Cook the fava beans, stirring occasionally, until they begin to break down, about 15 to 30 minutes depending on the starchiness of the beans. If necessary, add more water.

Bring a large pot of salted water to a boil and cook the bucatini, following the directions on the package, until barely al dente. Drain, reserving 1 cup of pasta water. Return the pasta to the pot and add the fava bean sauce. Add a splash of pasta water and bring to a simmer. Cook until the sauce reduces and clings to the pasta. Add more pasta water if needed.

Add the Parmigiano and olive oil, season to taste. Top with grated Pecorino-Romano and some freshly ground black pepper.

PER SERVING: 575 CALORIES, 19.34G FAT, 77.37G CARBS, 20.08G PROTEIN, 2.95G FIBER, 86MG CALCIUM, 4.03MG IRON, 271MG SODIUM, 291µG FOLATE

bucatini amatriciana with bacon

Iron Chef and supermom Cat Cora kindly customized this—her number-one pregnancy-craving recipe from her cookbook *Classics with a Twist*—for the pregnant palate. She couldn't get enough spiciness, tomatoes, and pasta, and once you try this recipe, you may feel the same. When buying ingredients, look for pancetta or guanciale that is nitrate-free; it's more healthful for your baby.

Serves 6

½ pound unsmoked pancetta or guanciale
(nitrate-free), sliced thinly and
finely chopped
1 large yellow onion, halved and sliced
(about 1½ cups)
4 cloves garlic, minced
1 teaspoon red pepper flakes, plus
more to taste
1 cup canned tomato sauce
1 cup crushed tomatoes
1 tablespoon chopped fresh oregano
kosher salt and freshly ground
black pepper
1 pound bucatini
freshly grated Pecorino-Romano

Bring a large pot of salted water to a boil. Line a platter with paper towels.

In a sauté pan, cook the guanciale over medium heat just until the fat is rendered and the pieces are beginning to crisp. Transfer to the paper towels to drain.

Pour the fat from the skillet, reserving 2 tablespoons. Add the onion and sauté until brown, 5 to 6 minutes. Add the garlic and red pepper flakes and sauté just until the garlic is lightly browned and aromatic, about 2 minutes. Add the tomato sauce and the crushed tomatoes. Reduce the heat to low, add the oregano, salt, and pepper and let simmer until the sauce thickens, 15 to 20 minutes.

Meanwhile, break the bucatini in half and cook, following directions on the package. Drain, reserving 1 cup of pasta water. Return the pasta back to the pot and add the sauce. Toss to combine, and add a little of the reserved pasta water if the pasta isn't saucy enough. Top with freshly grated pecorino cheese and serve immediately.

PER SERVING: 480 CALORIES, 16.15G FAT, 64.49G CARBS, 16.77G PROTEIN, 2.46G FIBER, 71MG CALCIUM, 3.36MG IRON, 225MG SODIUM, 242µG FOLATE

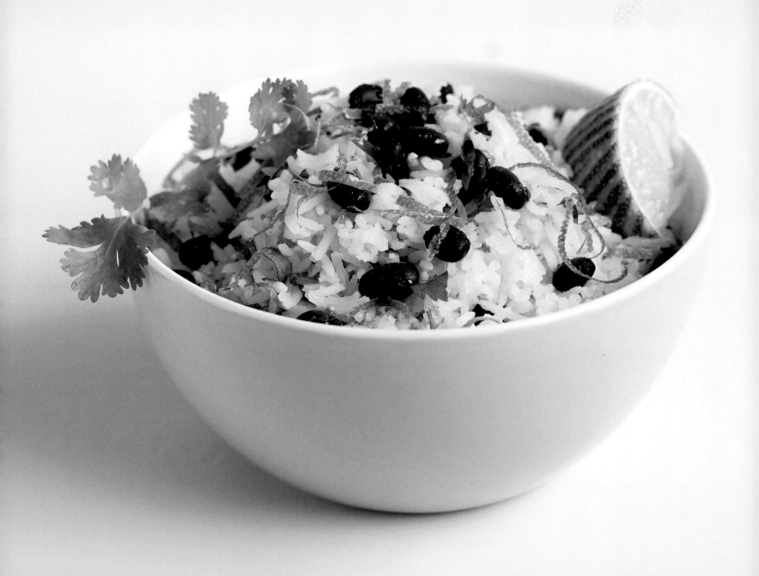

chapter six

sides

braised brussels sprouts with bacon

grilled vegetables

Forget everything you think about Brussels sprouts—except for, perhaps, that they can cause a wee extra flatulence, which is true. This preparation—flavored with bacon and chicken broth—will make even haters into lovers of these adorable bite-size heads of cabbage.

It's easy to forget that sometimes the simplest recipe makes the best food. And grilled vegetables is a reason to remember that. Naturally savory and sweet—due to the caramelizing that happens during the grilling process—filling, healthy, and exceptionally tasty, they can be served solo, between two slices of bread, or diced, tossed, and served as a salad.

Serves 4

12 Brussels sprouts
kosher salt
1 thick-cut slice nitrate-free bacon
¼ cup chicken broth
¼ teaspoon lemon juice

Serves 4

3 tablespoons olive oil, plus more for oiling grill
1 garlic clove, pressed or minced
1 teaspoon kosher salt
pinch freshly ground black pepper
2 zucchini, halved lengthwise
1 red bell pepper, cored, seeded, and quartered
1 orange bell pepper, cored, seeded, and quartered
1 eggplant, sliced into ½-inch disks and salted
5 sprigs fresh basil, for garnish (optional)

Trim the ends off the Brussels sprouts and remove and discard any discolored outer leaves.

Bring a large pot of salted water to a boil. Add the sprouts and cook until crunchy, but tender, about 5 minutes. Drain, let cool, and slice the sprouts in half through the stem.

In a large sauté pan over medium heat, cook the bacon until it begins to brown. Add the Brussels sprouts, cut-sides down, in one layer, and cook until brown, about 4 minutes. Combine the chicken stock and lemon juice in a liquid measuring cup, add them to the pan, and cook until the liquid has just evaporated. Serve.

Lightly oil and preheat the grill.

In a mixing bowl, mix the olive oil, garlic, salt, and pepper. Baste both sides of each vegetable with the garlic olive oil.

Grill the vegetables over a low flame until tender and lightly charred on each side, approximately 8 to 10 minutes for the peppers and 8 minutes for the zucchini and eggplant. Arrange the vegetables on a platter, garnish with the fresh basil, and serve warm or at room temperature.

PER SERVING: 40 CALORIES, 1.04G FAT, 5.69G CARBS, 3.05G PROTEIN, 2.17G FIBER, 24MG CALCIUM, 0.86MG IRON, 81MG SODIUM, 35µG FOLATE

PER SERVING: 157 CALORIES, 10.21 FAT, 14.97G CARBS, 3.21G PROTEIN, 7.02G FIBER, 32MG CALCIUM, 1.02MG IRON, 595MG SODIUM, 85µG FOLATE

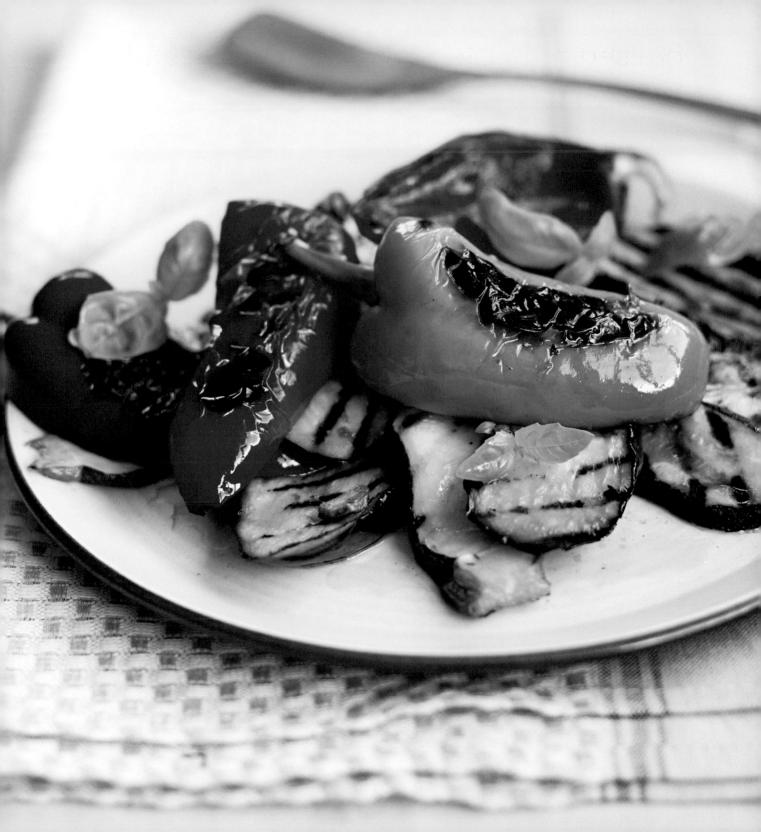

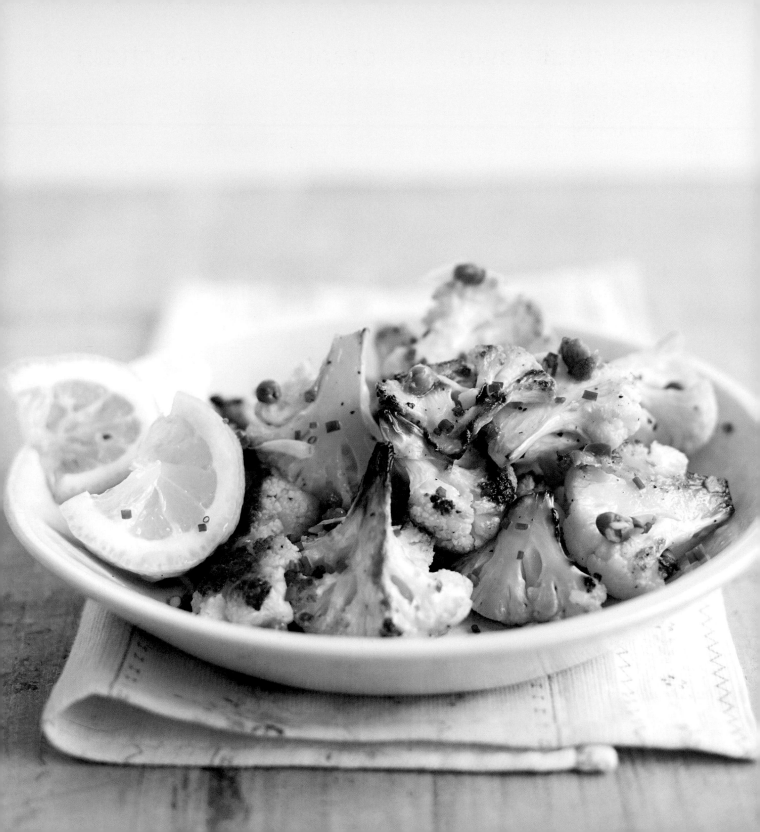

roasted cauliflower with caper vinaigrette

Even if you think you don't like cauliflower, you've got to try this recipe. Absurdly easy to make, it has robust flavor that belies its healthy attributes. In fact, the flavor is so good on its own, you might even want to skip the dressing (and its extra calories). Regardless, you can dine with the confidence that cauliflower is a good source of protein, dietary fiber, vitamins C, K, B6, and folate.

Serves 4

2 tablespoons extra-virgin olive oil
¼ teaspoon kosher salt
pinch freshly ground black pepper
1 (2½-to 3-pound) head cauliflower, cut into florets
2 garlic cloves, peeled
1 tablespoon capers, drained and minced
1 teaspoon fresh lemon juice

Preheat the oven to 450°F and place the rack in the lower third of the oven.

In a mixing bowl, combine 1 tablespoon olive oil, salt, and pepper. Add the cauliflower and garlic cloves and toss until evenly coated. Transfer the mixture to a rimmed baking sheet and roast, turning once, until golden and just tender, about 25 minutes.

Transfer the cauliflower to a serving bowl and set aside. Transfer the roasted garlic cloves to a small mixing bowl with the capers and mash them together. Whisk in the lemon juice and remaining 1 tablespoon olive oil.

Drizzle the dressing over the cauliflower, and serve.

PER SERVING: 114 CALORIES, 6.73G FAT, 11.88G CARBS, 4.32G PROTEIN, 5.137G FIBER, 49MG CALCIUM, 1.04MG IRON, 271MG SODIUM, 119µG FOLATE

creamed swiss chard

Anyone who loves creamed spinach will be smitten with this creamy, rich dish loaded with vitamins, minerals, and daily fiber. You can make it up to a day ahead and refrigerate it until ready to serve.

Serves 4

2 teaspoons extra-virgin olive oil
½ cup chopped yellow onion
2 bunches Swiss chard leaves, chopped (about 6 cups packed)
⅓ cup water
½ cup low-fat milk
1 tablespoon flour
generous pinch ground nutmeg
½ teaspoon kosher salt
freshly ground black pepper

Heat the olive oil in a large saucepan over medium heat. Add the onion and cook until translucent but not browned, 3 to 4 minutes. Add the chard and ⅓ cup water and cook, covered but stirring occasionally, until tender, 4 minutes.

In a small saucepan, heat the milk over medium heat until hot and whisk in the flour and nutmeg until blended. Stir until the sauce thickens, 3 to 5 minutes. Pour the milk mixture into the Swiss chard, add the salt and pepper, to taste, stir, and serve immediately.

PER SERVING: 161 CALORIES, 3.45G FAT, 24.53G CARBS, 5.25G PROTEIN, 4.17G FIBER, 59MG CALCIUM, 3.14MG IRON, 309MG SODIUM, 81µG FOLATE

sautéed spinach with garlic and lemon

A lighter, cleaner-flavored alternative to the ever-comforting Creamed Swiss Chard (page 119), this ultra-healthy side dish is a perfect accompaniment to grilled meats, including Grilled Herbed Chicken (page 102).

Serves 4

2 teaspoons extra-virgin olive oil
½ teaspoon minced fresh garlic
10 ounces fresh baby spinach
kosher salt
4 lemon wedges

Heat the oil in a large sauté pan over medium heat. Add the garlic and sauté it until pale golden, about 1 minute. Add the spinach and cook, stirring occasionally, until wilted, about 3 minutes.

Season with salt and serve with lemon wedges on the side.

PER SERVING: 58 CALORIES, 2.51G FAT, 14.24G CARBS, 3.34G PROTEIN, 6.64G FIBER, 136MG CALCIUM, 2.70MG IRON, 640MG SODIUM, 137µG FOLATE

lime rice with black beans and cilantro

A gorgeous accompaniment to grilled chicken or fish or a perfect base for a "dinner bowl" of cubed grilled chicken or steak, chopped romaine lettuce, and salsa, this pretty and lively side dish transforms everyday rice into tangy, exciting goodness. It also provides a decent dose of protein, folate, and dietary fiber.

Serves 4

1½ cups canned black beans
1 teaspoon vegetable oil
1 teaspoon butter
½ teaspoon minced fresh garlic
⅔ cup white basmati rice
1 cup water
½ teaspoon kosher salt
1 tablespoon fresh lime juice
⅛ teaspoon fresh lime zest
1 tablespoon fresh chopped cilantro

Drain, rinse, and strain the black beans to remove excess moisture. Set aside.

In a large heavy saucepan over low heat, heat the oil and butter until hot but not smoking. Stir in the garlic and sauté for 2 minutes, stirring frequently. Stir in the rice. Add the water, salt, lime juice, and lime zest, bring to a boil, cover, then simmer over low heat for 20 minutes.

Fluff the rice with a fork, and gently mix in the cilantro and black beans. Serve.

PER SERVING: 216 CALORIES, 2.45G FAT, 40.39G CARBS, 7.97G PROTEIN, 6.04G FIBER, 28MG CALCIUM, 2.70MG IRON, 447MG SODIUM, 167µG FOLATE

oven-roasted parmesan french fries

These delightfully crispy, Parmesan-sprinkled, oven-roasted potatoes are almost as satisfying as their fryer-immersed friends—especially when dipped into your favorite condiment. After all, what are French fries but gorgeously greasy vehicles for ketchup, aioli, or gravy? Make these to satisfy your fries craving and you'll feel a little less guilty when you reach for seconds. And if you're a traditionalist, skip the cheese.

Serves 4

4 large unpeeled russet potatoes, washed, dried, and sliced into ½-inch wedges
1 tablespoon plus 1½ teaspoons canola oil
1 teaspoon kosher salt
3 tablespoons finely grated Parmesan

Preheat the oven to 450°F. Line a baking sheet with parchment paper.

In a large bowl, toss the potato wedges in oil until well coated. Spread the potatoes in a single layer on the lined baking sheet and sprinkle generously with salt. Roast for 15 minutes, turn the wedges over, and continue roasting until browned and crisp.

Remove the fries from the oven, toss in a bowl with the Parmesan, and serve hot or at room temperature.

PER SERVING: 376 CALORIES, 7.75G FAT, 64.45G CARBS, 11.68G PROTEIN, 6.88G FIBER, 180MG CALCIUM, 3.32MG IRON, 794MG SODIUM, 78µG FOLATE

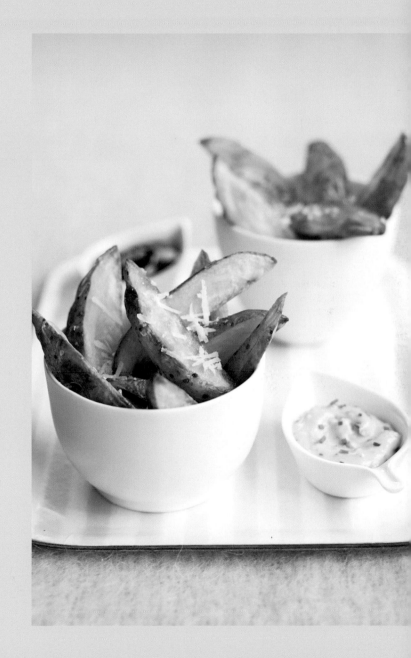

chinese-style green beans

Sometimes called "dry-braised," these stir-fried string beans have such robust flavor—thanks to the ginger, garlic, and soy sauce—that they make a deeply satisfying meal, especially if paired with a little rice. Want to add extra kick? Throw some chile paste or red pepper flakes into the mix during cooking.

Serves 4

2 teaspoons vegetable oil
1 pound green beans or Chinese long beans, ends trimmed
1 tablespoon chopped garlic
1 tablespoon chopped ginger
¼ cup finely chopped scallions
1 tablespoon soy sauce

Heat 1 teaspoon oil in a wok or large sauté pan over medium-high heat. Add the green beans and stir-fry, stirring frequently, until they start to shrivel and brown, about 7 minutes.

Transfer the beans to a paper towel-lined plate. Increase the heat to high and add the remaining teaspoon of oil, the garlic, ginger, and scallions. Stir-fry for a few seconds.

Add the green beans and the soy sauce, stir, and serve warm.

PER SERVING: 63 CALORIES, 2.35G FAT, 9.76G CARBS, 2.81G PROTEIN, 4.13G FIBER, 50MG CALCIUM, 1.42MG IRON, 259MG SODIUM, 46µG FOLATE

quinoa tabbouleh

This spin on the classic Middle Eastern salad, "tabbouleh," swaps traditionally used bulgur wheat (which you could also use) for nutritional superstar quinoa, which is high in "complete protein," meaning that it includes all nine essential amino acids. Serve it as a dinner side dish or store it covered in the refrigerator for a healthy and filling go-to snack.

Serves 4

1 tablespoon extra-virgin olive oil
¼ cup fresh squeezed lemon juice
½ teaspoon kosher salt
pinch freshly ground pepper
2 cups cooked quinoa
½ cup seeded and finely diced tomatoes
½ cup peeled and diced cucumber
1 cup finely chopped flat-leaf parsley
½ cup minced scallions, white and green parts
3 tablespoons slivered fresh mint leaves, plus whole leaves for garnish

In a small bowl or cup, combine the olive oil, lemon juice, salt, and pepper. Set aside.

In a serving bowl, toss together the quinoa, tomatoes, cucumber, parsley, scallions, and mint. Add the dressing, toss until evenly coated, and serve.

PER SERVING: 161 CALORIES, 3.45G FAT, 24.53G CARBS, 5.25G PROTEIN, 4.17G FIBER, 59MG CALCIUM, 3.14MG IRON, 309MG SODIUM, 81µG FOLATE

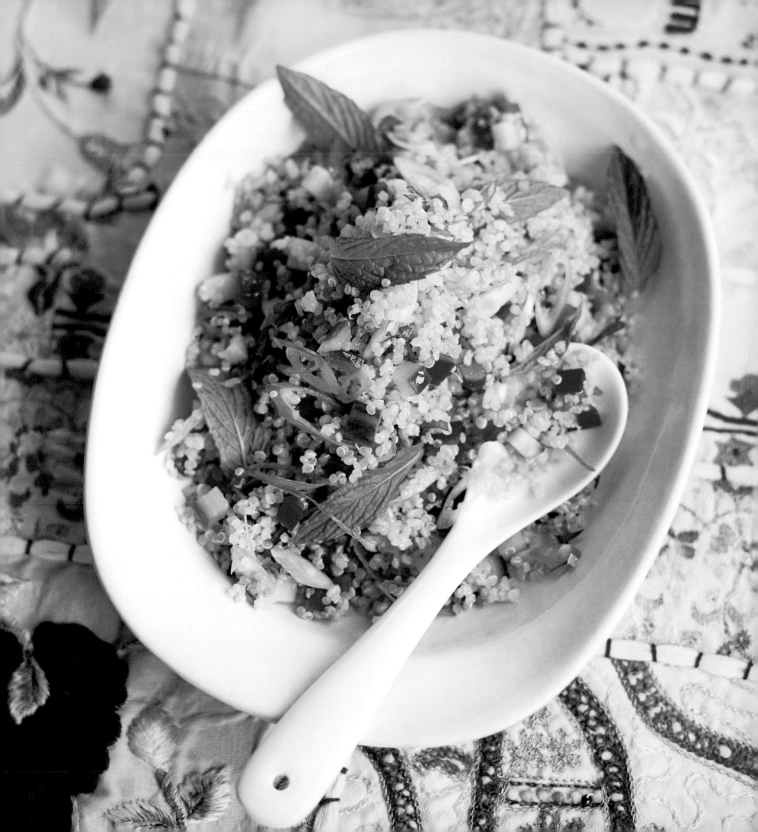

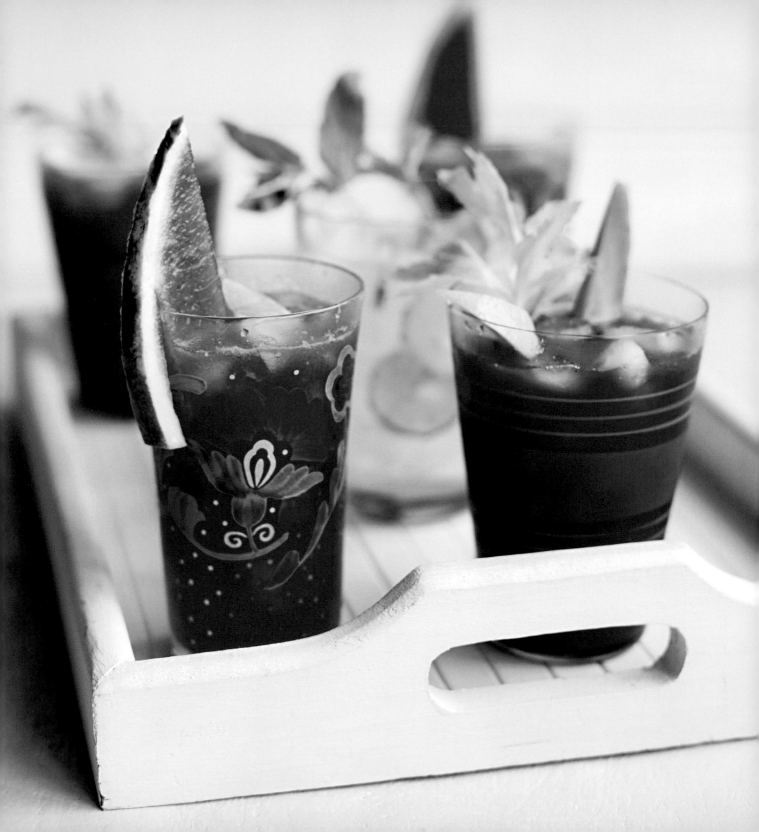

desserts & beverages

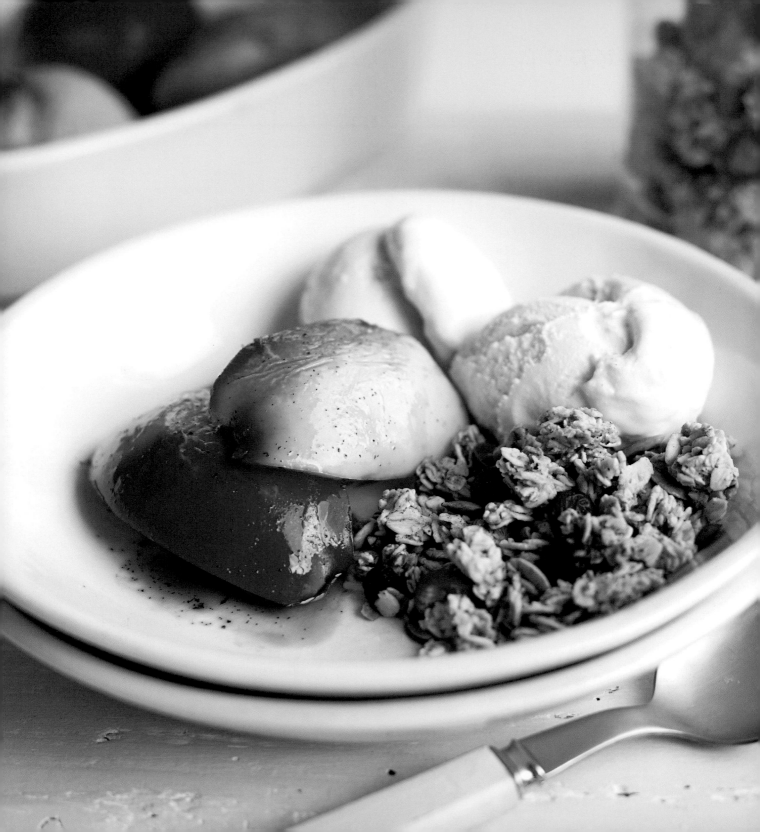

baked apple à la mode

You can treat yourself to a sizable dessert while only putting a small dent in the ice cream carton if you partake in this heaven-scented baked dessert. Or skip the ice cream altogether and you've got a great breakfast.

Serves 4

2 large Golden Delicious apples, halved and cored
¼ cup apple juice
1 teaspoon fresh lemon juice
¼ teaspoon vanilla extract
⅓ teaspoon ground cinnamon
1 heaping tablespoon raisins (optional)
1 cup vanilla ice cream
2 tablespoons granola (see page 32, or store-bought)

Preheat oven to 325°F.

Place the apples, cut sides down, in a baking dish just large enough to contain the apples.

In a bowl, combine the apple juice, lemon juice, vanilla, and cinnamon and pour the mixture around the apples. Bake the apples until they are soft, occasionally basting, about 20 minutes. Cool slightly.

Spoon the apple halves, ¼ cup ice cream, and ½ tablespoon granola, and serve immediately.

PER SERVING: 140 CALORIES, 2.67G FAT, 28.93G CARBS, 1.68G PROTEIN, 3.48G FIBER, 35MG CALCIUM, 0.47MG IRON, 16MG SODIUM, 7µG FOLATE

banana "ice cream" with caramel and toasted walnuts

Believe it or not, you can have your ice cream and eat it too—if you use this surprising recipe, which miraculously transforms your basic banana (loaded with fiber, vitamins C and B6, potassium, and manganese) into gelato-like decadence. Seriously. With nary a hint of sugar, eggs, or cream in the "ice cream," you can guiltlessly add a sprinkle of toasted shredded coconut or a drizzle of chocolate or caramel without indulging in too many empty calories. There's no need to hold back on the toasted walnuts, either; they're an excellent source of omega-3 fatty acids.

Serves 4

4 frozen peeled bananas
4 tablespoons toasted or raw walnuts
4 teaspoons store-bought chocolate or caramel sauce

Slice the bananas into ½-inch-thick discs. Put them in a blender on the slowest speed until they become little bits. Stop and scrape down the sides. Repeat several times until the banana begins forming a creamy, gelato-like ball.

Blend until smooth, spoon into four dessert bowls, and top each with a tablespoon of walnuts and a teaspoon of sauce.

PER SERVING: 174 CALORIES, 5.32G FAT, 31.94G CARBS, 2.69G PROTEIN, 3.74G FIBER, 14MG CALCIUM, 0.60MG IRON, 22MG SODIUM, 30µG FOLATE

banana coconut cream crumbles

Crunchy on top, smooth and creamy in the middle, and lighter than it looks and tastes, this glorious dessert is a fine source of dietary fiber, vitamins B6 and C, and potassium. It's also elegant enough to impress company with minimal effort.

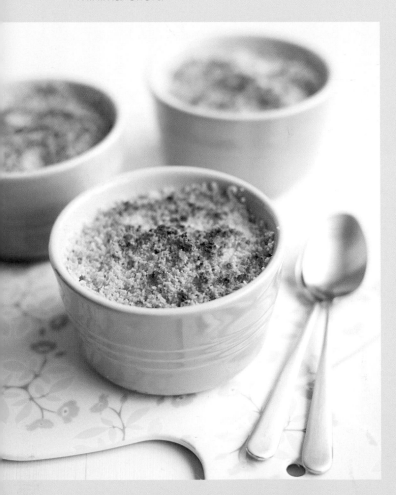

Serves 4

8 teaspoons sugar
1½ tablespoons cornstarch
⅜ teaspoon salt
½ cup low-fat milk
¾ cup light coconut milk
½ large egg
½ teaspoon vanilla extract
¼ cup all-purpose flour
¼ cup almonds, ground into a coarse meal
   (use a coffee grinder or food processor)
¼ cup firmly packed light brown sugar
2½ tablespoons unsalted butter, cut into ½-inch pieces
2 ripe bananas

In a small bowl, whisk together the sugar, cornstarch, and ¼ teaspoon salt.

Bring the milk and coconut milk to a simmer in a medium heavy saucepan. Gradually add the sugar mixture, stirring constantly. Gradually whisk in the egg. Stir over medium heat until the mixture boils and thickens, about 5 minutes. Remove from the heat, mix in the vanilla, and set aside.

In a mixing bowl, combine the flour, almond meal, brown sugar, ⅛ teaspoon salt, and butter and mix until the butter becomes the size of small peas. Set aside.

Preheat the broiler. Slice the banana into ¼-inch-thick slices. Layer the bottoms of four oven-safe ramekins with banana slices. Top with ¼ cup coconut pudding. Crumble the butter-almond topping mixture on top of the pudding so that it covers the pudding entirely. Place the individual servings under the broiler until the crumbly tops are golden brown, about 3 minutes. Serve immediately.

PER SERVING: 329 CALORIES, 16.77G FAT, 42.60G CARBS, 5.32G PROTEIN, 2.58G FIBER, 85 MG CALCIUM, 2.18MG IRON, 250MG SODIUM, 24µG FOLATE

raspberry turnovers

As decadent as turnovers found in your favorite bakery—complete with gooey fruit filling wrapped in a flaky, buttery crust—these homemade versions use less puff pastry and provide less calories without losing any of the flavor. Plus, raspberries include great dietary fiber, vitamin C, and manganese.

Serves 4

butter for greasing pan
2 cups fresh raspberries
1 tablespoon water, plus more for puff pastry
4½ teaspoons sugar
2 teaspoons lemon juice
1½ teaspoons cornstarch
4 (3 x 3-inch) pieces of puff pastry, thawed but chilled

Preheat the oven to 400°F. Grease a baking sheet with butter.

Place the berries, 4 teaspoons sugar, and water into a saucepan over medium heat and cook, stirring frequently, until the berries break down. Add the lemon juice and cornstarch and stir until the berry mixture thickens, about 3 minutes. Set aside.

Stretch out each piece of puff pastry to 4 inches square and place them on the prepared baking sheet. Place ¼ of the raspberry mixture in the center, leaving ¾ inches of dough on each side. Using a pastry brush, dampen the dough with water. Fold the dough in half diagonally, over the filling. Press the edges to seal and crimp them with a fork. Brush the top of each turnover with water and sprinkle evenly with the remaining sugar. Chill in the refrigerator for 20 to 30 minutes.

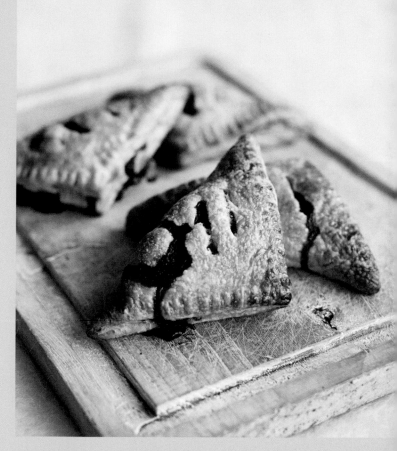

With the tip of a paring knife, cut three small slits in the top of each pastry. Bake in the center of the oven for 15 minutes, or until the pastry is golden. Serve warm.

PER SERVING: 210 CALORIES, 10.53G FAT, 25.99G CARBS, 2.82G PROTEIN, 4.44G FIBER, 18MG CALCIUM, 1.16MG IRON, 71MG SODIUM, 35µG FOLATE

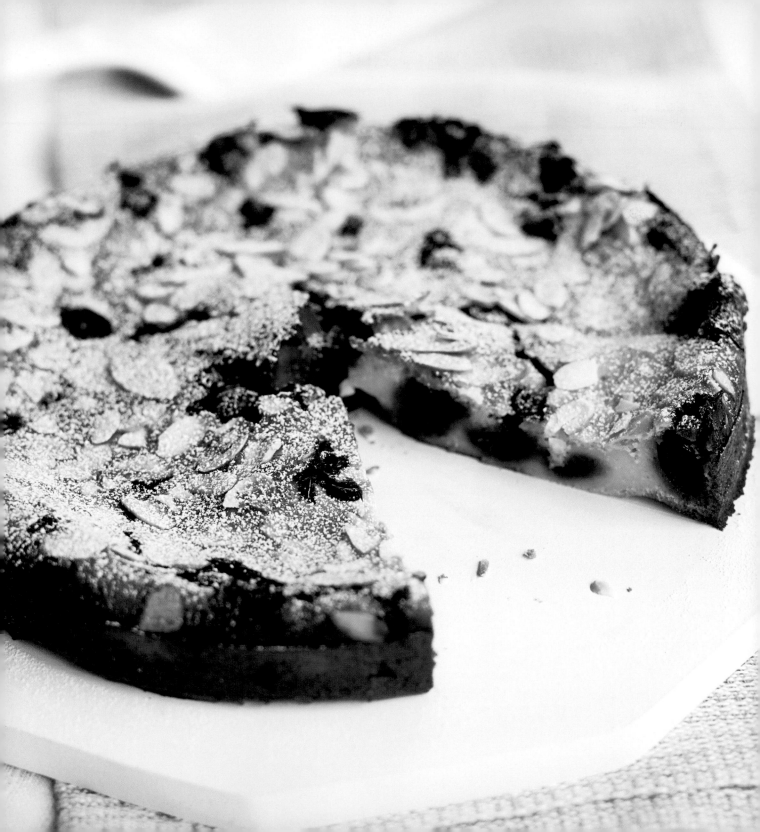

anise-kissed blueberry and almond clafouti

"Clafouti" is a pancake-custard hybrid made of fruit and a cake batter. In this case, the result is an antioxidant-rich blueberry bonanza surrounded by a thin but deliciously dense and creamy layer of cake. Don't be afraid to substitute other fruits—pear or plum slices or cherry halves would also be excellent. And if you're concerned with overeating, you can bake the berries and batter in cupcake trays (just be sure to cook them for a shorter time). Finally, use organic blueberries; their non-organic counterparts are one of the highest pesticide-contaminated fruits on the market.

Serves 6

½ cup raw almonds
1 cup low-fat milk
¾ teaspoon butter for greasing
1 cup fresh or frozen blueberries
2 large eggs, room temperature
1 teaspoon almond extract
1 teaspoon anise-flavored liqueur
¼ teaspoon kosher salt
⅓ cup sugar
6 tablespoons all-purpose flour
¼ cup sliced almonds
½ teaspoon powdered sugar

Process the whole almonds in a food processor until finely ground; do not over-process or they will become pasty. Transfer to a small saucepan, add the milk, and bring it to simmer. Remove the almond milk from the heat and let sit for 30 minutes.

Pour the milk through a fine-mesh strainer, pressing the almond bits to extract all the liquid. Discard the solids and set aside.

Preheat oven to 375°F. Butter an 8-inch baking pan and scatter the berries along the bottom.

Whisk the eggs, almond extract, liqueur, salt, and sugar until well blended. Add the almond milk and whisk to blend. Sift the flour into the mixture and beat until smooth. Pour the mixture over the blueberries in the baking pan, top with the sliced almonds, and bake until set and a knife inserted into the center comes out clean, about 30 minutes.

Cool, lightly dust with powdered sugar, and serve warm or at room temperature.

PER SERVING: 226 CALORIES, 9.67G FAT, 26.96G CARBS, 7.81G PROTEIN, 2.72G FIBER, 101MG CALCIUM, 1.07MG IRON, 138MG SODIUM, 20µG FOLATE

angel food cake with pineapple compôte

A blend of the light lusciousness of angel food cake and the moist, sweet-tangy goodness of pineapple upside-down cake, this recipe allows you to feel like you're really indulging—without going too far down a decadent path. Incidentally, you can swap pineapple for strawberries or peaches or both (with orange-peel strands, as shown at right), or skip fruit altogether and add two teaspoons grated lime, orange, or lemon zest to infuse a citrus flavor into the cake. Bonus: You can freeze any extra cake in plastic-wrapped single servings, with pineapple separately, for future cravings.

Serves 12

1½ cups room-temperature egg whites (from about 12 large eggs)
1 teaspoon vanilla extract
1 teaspoon cream of tartar
¾ cup sugar
¾ cup cake flour, sifted
¼ teaspoon plus 1 pinch kosher salt
1 tablespoon butter
½ cup brown sugar
1 cup crushed canned pineapple in unsweetened pineapple juice, strained

Position a rack in the center of the oven and preheat to 350°F.

In a large bowl, beat the egg whites and vanilla on medium speed with an electric mixer until frothy. Add the cream of tartar and beat at high speed until soft peaks form. Gradually add the sugar, beating until stiff peaks form.

Mix the flour and salt in a small bowl. Sprinkle ⅓ of the flour mixture over the egg whites and gently fold in until incorporated. Repeat with the remaining flour mixture, a third at a time. Gently spoon the batter into an ungreased tube pan. Bake the cake for 35 minutes, or until the cake springs to the touch and a wooden skewer comes out clean when you stick it into the center. Let the cake cool upside down on a wire rack for 1 hour or more.

Meanwhile, in a small saucepan over medium heat, add the butter and brown sugar and stir until the butter melts. Add the pineapple and a generous pinch of kosher salt. Set aside.

Gently remove the cake from the pan, slice it, then serve with a heaping tablespoon of pineapple compote.

PER SERVING: 136 CALORIES, 0.95G FAT, 28.05G CARBS, 4.11G PROTEIN, 0.36G FIBER, 11MG CALCIUM, 0.75MG IRON, 100MG SODIUM, 17µG FOLATE

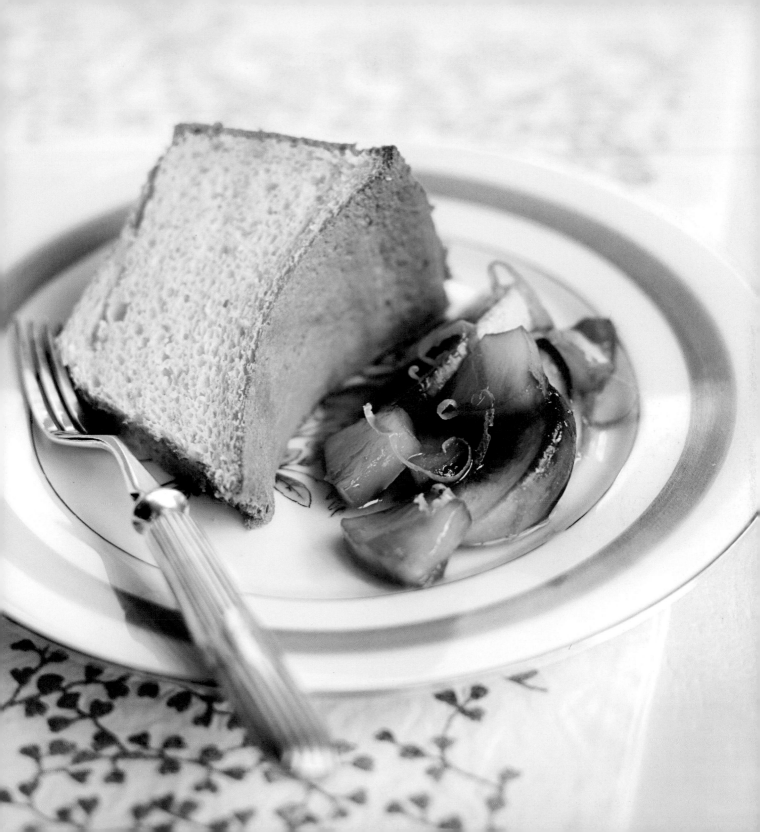

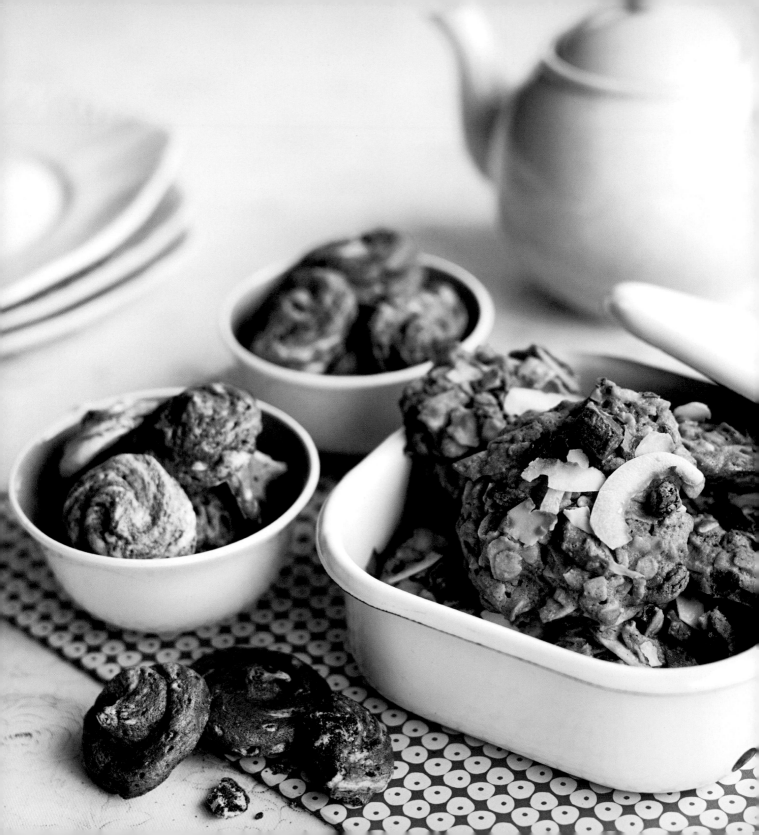

chocolate coconut oatmeal cookies

Moist yet crisp on the edges, these cookies promise cholesterol-fighting fiber, folic acid, and essential fatty acids—not to mention exceptional flavor. Add dried currants or cranberries, raisins, almond or pecan bits for even more pizzazz.

Makes 24 cookies

½ cup (1 stick) unsalted butter, at room temperature
½ cup lightly packed dark brown sugar
1 large egg, at room temperature
1 teaspoon vanilla extract
¾ cup all-purpose flour
½ teaspoon baking powder
½ teaspoon ground cinnamon
½ teaspoon kosher salt
½ cup sweetened coconut flakes
1½ cups old-fashioned oats
¼ cup semisweet chocolate chips

Preheat the oven to 350°F. Line a baking sheet with parchment paper.

In a large bowl, beat the butter and brown sugar until fluffy. Mix in the egg and vanilla until well combined.

Sift the flour, baking powder, cinnamon, and salt together into a bowl and then fold into the butter mixture. Mix in the coconut, oats, and chocolate chips until just combined.

Drop heaping tablespoons of the batter, 1 inch apart, onto the baking sheet (or use a pastry bag to make the more traditional swirl-shaped cookies). Bake for 15 minutes, until golden. Cool completely before serving.

PER COOKIE: 120 CALORIES, 5.55G FAT, 14.64G CARBS, 2.53G PROTEIN, 1.37G FIBER, 17MG CALCIUM, 0.68MG IRON, 68MG SODIUM, 8µG FOLATE

ultra-chocolate meringue cookies

Crisp melt-in-your-mouth texture, rich brownie-like flavor, and astoundingly low calories make these light-as-air, two-bite cookies a nearly perfect partner for the pregnant chocoholic. The fact that egg whites are a solid source of protein seals the deal.
Tip: To avoid eating them all in one sitting, store extra cookies in a container for up to two months.

Makes approximately 30 cookies

3 egg whites
⅛ teaspoon kosher salt
⅛ teaspoon cream of tartar
½ teaspoon vanilla extract (or peppermint extract)
⅓ cup sugar
¼ cup unsweetened cocoa powder

Preheat oven to 225°F. Line 2 baking sheets with aluminum foil.

In a large glass bowl, beat the egg whites, salt, cream of tartar, and vanilla until soft peaks form. Gradually add the sugar, beating until stiff peaks form. Sift in the cocoa powder, then gently fold in until incorporated.

Drop heaping teaspoonfuls of the batter, 1 inch apart, onto the baking sheets. Bake for 1¾ hours. Cool completely. Store the cookies in a cool, dry place.

PER COOKIE: 12 CALORIES, 0.09G FAT, 2.68G CARBS, 0.50G PROTEIN, 0.24G FIBER, 1MG CALCIUM, 0.10MG IRON, 15MG SODIUM, 0µG FOLATE

watermelon-yogurt granita

Watermelon is not only refreshing, it's also a favorite go-to fruit for fighting morning sickness, and is a natural diuretic, which means it battles bloated bellies. Plus, it tastes great.

Serves 4

6 cups 1-inch watermelon chunks, chilled,
   plus 4 small watermelon wedges
3 tablespoons sugar
¼ cup lemon juice
2 cups low-fat or nonfat plain Greek yogurt

In a food processor or blender, puree the watermelon chunks with the sugar, lemon juice, and yogurt. Pour into a shallow container and freeze for 1 hour.

Using a fork, stir the granita, breaking up any solid parts with the back of the fork. Freeze again until firm, about 2 to 3 hours, scraping the mixture with a fork every 30 minutes to form ice crystals.

Transfer to 4 dessert bowls, garnish with a watermelon wedge, and serve.

PER SERVING: 262 CALORIES, 0.74G FAT, 58.90G CARBS, 10.21G PROTEIN, 2.12G FIBER, 280MG CALCIUM, 1.35MG IRON, 99MG SODIUM, 31µG FOLATE

lemon rosemary pops

In aromatherapy, rosemary is used to battle fatigue. In this refreshing recipe, it's used to perk up both the spirit and the palate. Meanwhile, the tang of lemon quells the very common craving for citrus, and the ice-cold nature of a pop cools down the ever-heated pregnant body.

Makes 8 pops

2 cups water
3 fresh 4-inch rosemary sprigs
¼ cup sugar
½ cup lemon juice

In a medium saucepan, combine the water and rosemary. Bring to a simmer, stirring occasionally. Remove from the heat, stir in the sugar until it has dissolved, cover, and let the ingredients infuse for 10 minutes.

Add the lemon juice, stir, and strain into popsicle molds. Freeze until completely frozen, 2 to 3 hours. Enjoy!

PER POP: 28 CALORIES, 0.03G FAT, 7.70G CARBS, 0.08G PROTEIN, 0.15G FIBER, 4MG CALCIUM, 1.07MG IRON, 2MG SODIUM, 20µG FOLATE

strawberry-rhubarb pops

The sweet-sour combination of strawberry and rhubarb is frequently used in baked, crumble-topped desserts. But this version, based on a recipe by Massachusetts chef Jason Brown, moves the tangy, complementary flavors into fantastic frozen-dessert territory—with less fat and calories but just as much calcium, dietary fiber, and vitamin C. Note: You may need to use more or less sugar depending on the ripeness of the strawberries.

Makes 6

4 stalks rhubarb, cut into ½-inch pieces
   (about 2 cups)
1½ cups water
⅓ cup sugar
1 pint strawberries, washed, hulled, and halved
2 tablespoons lemon juice
pinch of kosher salt

Combine the rhubarb, water, sugar, and strawberries, and simmer, stirring frequently, until the rhubarb is extra-soft, about 20 minutes. Add the lemon juice and salt, transfer the mixture to a blender, and puree. Let cool. Pour the mixture into popsicle molds and freeze for at least 2 hours.

PER SERVING: 70 CALORIES, 0.19G FAT, 17.66G CARBS, 0.72G PROTEIN, 1.82G FIBER, 40MG CALCIUM, 0.32MG IRON, 52MG SODIUM, 17µG FOLATE

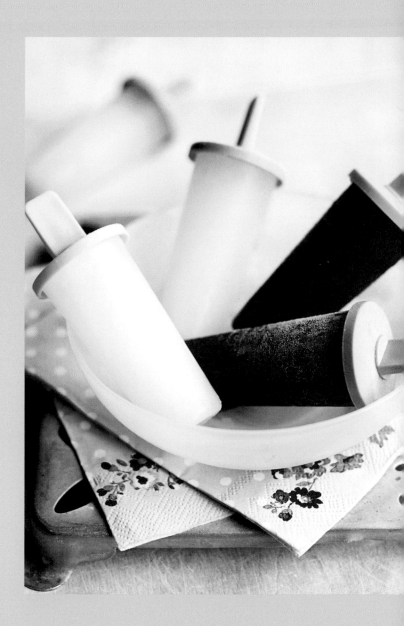

peanut butter-banana chocolate shake

A dessert and mini-meal, this rich, decadent drink by mom/athlete Jill Jackson, tastes as good as it sounds and provides protein, dietary fiber, and vitamin B6.

Serves 1

½ banana, peeled and frozen
½ cup nonfat milk
2 tablespoons peanut butter
1 tablespoon chocolate syrup

Combine all the ingredients in a blender and blend until smooth. Pour into a glass and enjoy.

PER SERVING: 333 CALORIES, 16.02G FAT, 38.02G CARBS, 13.19G PROTEIN, 3.94G FIBER, 170MG CALCIUM, 1.18MG IRON, 210MG SODIUM, 40µG FOLATE

blueberry-mango smoothie

Greek yogurt adds protein to this exceptional way to start the day.

Serves 1

½ cup apple juice
½ cup frozen or fresh mango pieces
½ fresh or frozen banana
⅛ cup frozen or fresh blueberries
¼ cup plain low-fat yogurt
1 teaspoon honey

Combine all the ingredients in a blender and blend until smooth. Pour into a glass and enjoy.

PER SERVING: 227 CALORIES, 0.54G FAT, 54.72G CARBS, 4.86G PROTEIN, 3.73G FIBER, 141 MG CALCIUM, 0.55MG IRON, 52MG SODIUM, 30µG FOLATE

warm vanilla milk

Whether you're in need of a soothing late-night snack or something to warm your soul, this gourmet version of a childhood favorite does the trick while providing you with vitamin D, riboflavin, and calcium. Plus, cinnamon is said to help with indigestion and nausea.

Serves 1

1 cup low-fat milk
1 teaspoon vanilla extract
2 teaspoons honey
1 dash cinnamon

Stir together the milk, vanilla, honey, and cinnamon in a small pot over medium heat. Warm until just hot. Serve warm.

PER SERVING: 172 CALORIES, 2.73G FAT, 26.01G CARBS, 9.73G PROTEIN, 0.20G FIBER, 352MG CALCIUM, 0.24MG IRON, 142MG SODIUM, 14µG FOLATE

citrus slushy

While a serious citrus craving may never be wholly satisfied, it can be temporarily abated with this cooling combo of frozen grapefruit and orange juice. Bonus: It delivers a nice dose of vitamin C. Tip: Make extra citrus ice cubes, keep them frozen, and whip up a slushy whenever you get the urge.

Serves 1

½ cup freshly squeezed grapefruit juice
½ cup freshly squeezed orange juice
2 teaspoons sugar (or more depending on the ripeness of the fruit)
½ cup water, plus more as needed

Combine all of the ingredients in a mixing bowl and stir until the sugar dissolves. Transfer to an ice tray and freeze until frozen, between 1 and 2 hours.

Place the frozen cubes in a blender with the water and blend until slushy, adding a little more water if necessary. Pour into a glass and drink with a straw for added fun.

PER SERVING: 135 CALORIES, 0.19G FAT, 32.66G CARBS, 1.49G PROTEIN, 0.37G FIBER, 24MG CALCIUM, 0.50MG IRON, 2MG SODIUM, 49µG FOLATE

ginger limeade

Frequently served hot or cold in the spas of Bali, Indonesia, this soothing concoction works wonders for morning sickness and gastrointestinal stress (thanks to the fresh ginger). It also tastes so good that you may want to remember the recipe for post-baby cocktail parties—adding white rum instantly transforms it into a sexy cocktail.

Serves 1

1 (¼ cup-size) piece of fresh ginger, peeled (about the size of a plum tomato)
½ cup water
⅛ cup honey
½ cup fresh lime juice

Grate the ginger on the finest holes of a box grater over a plate. Transfer all of the grated ginger (including from inside the grater) and ginger juice to a small saucepan. Add the water and bring to a boil.

Remove from the heat, stir in the honey until dissolved, and let cool. Pour the sweetened ginger juice through a fine-mesh strainer, pressing the pulp to squeeze out all the liquid. Discard the pulp. Add the lime juice to the ginger juice, stir until combined, and serve over ice.

PER SERVING: 44 CALORIES, 0.04G FAT, 12.34G CARBS, 0.27G PROTEIN, 0.26G FIBER, 5MG CALCIUM, 0.11MG IRON, 1MG SODIUM, 3µG FOLATE,

spa water

When pregnant, little things you can do to pamper yourself can really brighten your day. This recipe is case in point. An easy way to add subtle flavor, flair, and visual elegance to everyday water, it harkens the soothing, luxurious sentiment of a day spa.

Serves 6-8

½ lemon
½ lime
½ cucumber, peeled
½ cup muddled fresh mint

Slice the lemon and lime into ⅓-inch wheels and transfer to a pitcher. Add the cucumber and mint. Fill the pitcher with filtered water and refrigerate for at least 2 hours to let the flavors infuse.

PER SERVING: 8 CALORIES, 0.06G FAT, 2.31G CARBS, 0.46G PROTEIN, 1.08G FIBER, 21MG CALCIUM, 0.90MG IRON, 2MG SODIUM, 9µG FOLATE

tropical tease

You can forget ho-hum virgin options if you serve this drink at your next party. The exotic flavors of ginger, mango, and pomegranate enlivened with bubbly water turn the virgin cocktail into a celebratory affair. Plus you can easily add a shot of vodka or rum to each drink for those who are not in waiting.

Serves 1

3 fresh mint leaves
1 teaspoon-size piece of fresh ginger, peeled
3 tablespoons pomegranate concentrate
3 tablespoons mango juice
1 teaspoon fresh lemon juice
½ cup tonic

Muddle the mint leaves and ginger in a cocktail glass. Add the pomegranate concentrate, mango juice, and lemon juice, and stir to combine. Fill the glass with ice, top with tonic, and serve.

PER SERVING: 58 CALORIES, 0.22G FAT, 14.54G CARBS, 0.74G PROTEIN, 1.41G FIBER, 52MG CALCIUM, 2.27MG IRON, 35MG SODIUM, 31µG FOLATE

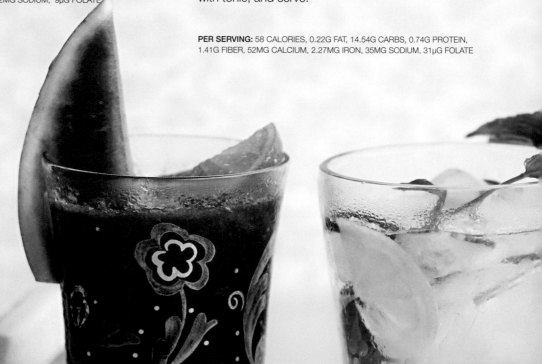

watermelon mamarita

Just because you're staving off alcohol doesn't mean you can't raise a glass in celebration. This virgin rendition of a watermelon margarita gives you good reason to toast. Created by award-winning bartender Jeff Burkhart, it has all the festivity of happy hour, minus the hangover—and it's made from watermelon, which is a natural diuretic and morning-sickness helper. Cheers!

Serves 1

1 to 1½ cups fresh seedless watermelon flesh
  (from about one large wedge)
2 tablespoons fresh lemon juice
juice of half a lime, plus 1 lime wedge
1 tablespoon agave nectar

Loosely fill a serving glass with ice. Transfer the ice to a blender. Add the watermelon, lemon juice, and lime juice and blend. Add the agave nectar, and continue blending until smooth. Taste. (You may need to adjust the lime juice, agave, or both.) Pour the mamarita back into the serving glass, garnish with the lime wedge, and serve.

PER SERVING: 119 CALORIES, 0.16G FAT, 33.19G CARBS, 1.19G PROTEIN, 1.04G FIBER, 16MG CALCIUM, 0.51MG IRON, 1MG SODIUM

mother mary

The genius behind the virgin Bloody Mary is that it can double as a mocktail and a wholesome drinkable meal—all the while imparting your body with ample amounts of vitamins A, C, and B6, folate, and potassium.

Serves 1

4 ounces tomato juice
1 teaspoon fresh lemon juice
½ teaspoon Worcestershire sauce
½ teaspoon prepared horseradish, or more to taste
2 drops Tabasco sauce
freshly ground black pepper
1 celery stalk
1 long, thin carrot stick

In a bowl or cocktail shaker, combine the tomato juice, lemon juice, Worcestershire sauce, horseradish, and Tabasco and mix well. Add pepper to taste. Fill a tall glass with ice, pour your Mary over the ice, and garnish with the celery and carrot.

PER SERVING: 28 CALORIES, 0.15G FAT, 7.34G CARBS, 1.21G PROTEIN, 1.08G FIBER, 24MG CALCIUM, 0.82MG IRON, 122MG SODIUM, 30µG FOLATE

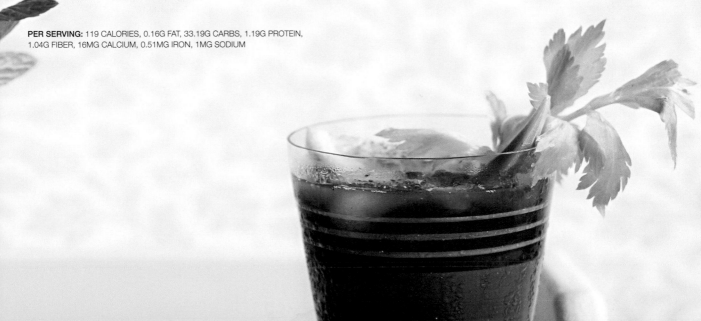

index